Alter Your Course
Parkinson's- The Early Years

Monique L. Giroux, MD
Medical Director and CEO
Movement & Neuroperformance Center Colorado
Medical Director of Movement Disorders & DBS Program at
Swedish Hospital, Englewood Colorado
Medical Director of Northwest Parkinson Foundation, Seattle
Washington
www.drgiroux.com

Sierra M. Farris, MA, MPAS, PA-C
Director Deep Brain Stimulation Services
Movement & Neuroperformance Center Colorado
Staff at Swedish Hospital, Englewood Colorado
www.dbsprogrammer.com

First Edition 2014

Part of the Movement & Neuroperformance Center of Colorado
Patient Empowerment Series ©2014

Movement & Neuroperformance Center Colorado, P.C.
499 E. Hampden Avenue, Suite 250 Englewood, Colorado 80113
Phone 303-781-0511; Fax 303-781-0517
www.centerformovement.org

Disclaimer: This content represents the opinions and experience of the authors and is for educational purposes only. This information should not be considered a substitute for medical professional advice or care and does not replace the advice of your physician. Readers should always discuss any information, questions or treatments with their medical providers. The authors do not accept any liability, loss, risk or complications that may be claimed or incurred as a consequence of the content of this book.

ISBN-13: 978-1497549647

ISBN-10: 1497549647

CONTENTS

INTRODUCTION

"You have Parkinson's disease." Sitting in your doctor's office, hearing these words for the first time, changes everything. You may not know much about Parkinson's disease (PD) or you may be familiar with PD through a family member or friend and wondering if your future will be similar to theirs. A normal reaction to the diagnosis is to question *"what changes are in store for me, how will this affect my future, or can I do anything that will make a difference in how I feel or progress."*

No one can predict the future. However, each of us can influence our future through the information we receive, attitudes we embrace and choices we make. As the title suggests, this book is written to give you the guidance, support and confidence you need to influence your future and *alter the course* of your life with Parkinson's disease.

We have spent almost two decades treating PD with a unique focus on both traditional and integrative medicine that includes holistic care, personal healing and emphasis on the patient experience. This has provided a lens for which to 'see' this condition with a different perspective -one with a focus on **what is possible instead of what is not possible**.

This book is not intended to be filled with facts about the disease; there are many books with this information. Instead we have focused on 2 questions, *"Does PD present an opportunity in disguise? What information, actions or attitudes are most helpful early in the disease to set the stage for living your best now and into the future?"*

Alter Your Course tells a different story- one that is emerging within you- the person with PD. Your story can be filled with hope, inspiration, empowerment, resiliency and strength.

Our patients have played a significant role in shaping the thoughts, guidance and information included in this book. For this reason, we have included actual patient care scenarios, many of which are probably already familiar and illustrate how thoughts, attitudes and actions are just as important as the medical or surgical therapies we prescribe. Each chapter concludes with advice designed to help you take control of your PD journey and *alter your course*. Most importantly, the last chapter is filled with advice; not from the authors, but people like you living with PD.

-Monique L. Giroux, MD

"Parkinson's changed my life. Not all for the worse and probably much more for the better. I now see and do things differently. I have learned to appreciate and focus on what is truly important in my life. My life is much richer because of the people PD has brought into my life. I exercise and take control of my health. I try to see the positive side of things." Steve, living with PD

DISEASE OVERVIEW

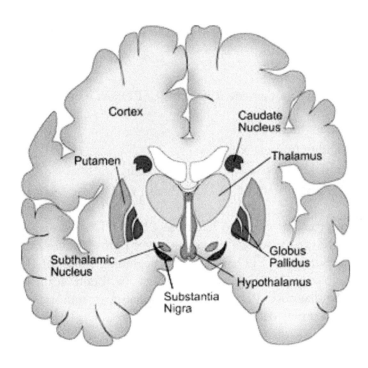

The basal ganglia, a collection of interconnected nerve cells affected in Parkinson's

Parkinson's disease is a brain condition associated with loss of nerve cells that produce the neurotransmitter dopamine in a region of the brain called the basal ganglia. The basal ganglia consist of an important network of cells or nuclei involved in planning, initiation and execution of movement. The main

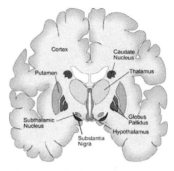

nuclei or interconnected cell regions are illustrated above. Loss of dopamine producing nerve cells occur in a nucleus called the substantia nigra. When dopamine levels reach low levels, symptoms emerge and slowly change how the body feels and moves.

Movement Disorder

The primary movement symptoms of PD can include:

- Resting tremor
- Rigidity (muscle stiffness)
- Bradykinesia (slowness of movement)
- Postural Instability (balance disturbance)

These symptoms are used to diagnose PD. A PD specialist will have a trained eye for the typical movement symptoms and are more likely to correctly diagnose PD earlier in the beginning stages of PD. Since we still do not have a laboratory test or brain scan that can definitively diagnose PD, seeing a specialist is important for an accurate and timely diagnosis.

Rest tremor is felt as a rhythmic shaking that is experienced when the arm or leg is resting or relaxed usually while sitting, lying down or walking. Rest tremor improves or disappears when you are moving that part of your body (unlike Essential or familial tremor which is a condition defined by tremor that worsens with active use of the arm or hands.) Rest tremor commonly worsens with stress or concentration. Rest tremor can be seen in the arms, legs, chin or lips. Internal tremor is a subclinical tremor (felt but not seen) often described as 'vibration' or even 'anxiousness' most often in the trunk or middle of the body.

Rigidity is described as a stiffness of the arms and/or legs in early PD. Stiffness is noted with movement and often associated with a feeling of heaviness, tightness or pain in the muscle and is associated with low levels of dopamine. The cause of the stiffness and or pain is very different than stiffness and pain associated with arthritis and therefore has a different treatment approach. *Cogwheel rigidity* describes ratchet- like movement that can be felt by your doctor at the wrist, elbow or knee when moving your arm or leg.

Bradykinesia means slowness of movement. Coupled with rigidity, bradykinesia causes trouble with speed of movement, initiating movement (taking a step) and performing sequential or repetitive movements like finger tapping.

Postural instability describes a problem with balance due to changes in the *righting reflex*. The righting reflex allows us to rapidly adjust our posture and stance to maintain balance when our center of gravity suddenly changes, such as when stepping off a curb or stumbling over an obstacle. This automatic response allows our brain to have finite control over the muscles of the body and respond to constant changes in position without falling. When the automatic reflex is diminished, people feel unsteady, cautious, may fall into walls or feel dizzy. Balance problems are a consequence of advanced PD and is not noted during early PD. If you are experiencing balance problems within the first few years of diagnosis, this may be due to other problems (such as peripheral neuropathy common in diabetes, inner ear problems, medication side effects, heart problems, and stroke) or atypical parkinsonism.

The following problems or observations are noted in early disease:

- Symptoms begin on one side of the body
- Decreased arm swing on one side when walking
- Decreased stride length or dragging your foot while walking
- Scuffing your toes, especially when tired
- Change in leg coordination when cycling or running
- Sense of muscle fatigue or heaviness in your arm or leg on one side of the body

- Difficulty completing repetitive movements due to sense of *'muscle fatigue'*
- Trouble with hand coordination especially on one side noted with bimanual tasks, i.e., shampooing
- Reduced range of motion in your shoulder, shoulder pain or frozen shoulder
- Masked like face or change in facial expression called *hypomimia*
- Decreased or small handwriting called *micrographia*

The following illustration is a handwriting sample of a person with Parkinson's disease. Note that letters are small, cramped and become even smaller over time. Analysis of handwriting can aid in the diagnosis of PD and is a visual representation of the symptoms described above.

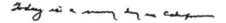

'Today is a sunny day in California.'

Preclinical Syndrome

Although we think of PD as a movement disorder, certain non-motor symptoms may actually precede movement problems. These problems in isolation are common and not specific to PD. However these problems can be the first signs of PD, beginning before movement problems emerge:

- Depression or anxiety- unexplained by other conditions or problems
- REM sleep disorder- vivid, active and physical dreaming such as yelling, kicking, punching and acting out of dreams during REM (rapid eye movement) sleep
- Reduced or loss of smell
- Constipation

As the presence of a preclinical syndrome suggests, PD begins years before the first movement symptoms and often many years before diagnosis. This is especially true for young onset PD (age of first symptoms less than 40-50 years) or people without tremor because diagnosis can be difficult in these situations.

As mentioned earlier, symptoms emerge after critical levels of dopamine cells are lost and dopamine levels are too low to sustain normal movement. Motor symptoms typically do not appear until over 60% of dopamine nerve cells are lost which shows us the brain and body have a tremendous ability to compensate and function despite dopamine nerve cell loss. Initially symptoms are mild, can be intermittent and can even be overcome with effort.

There are additional factors that influence exactly when symptoms begin to show. The following very common scenario is a patient story illustrating how personal factors influence the onset of symptoms:

"I first noted symptoms 15 years ago. My right thumb twitched for 3 days. It all started when I was attending a funeral for my father. Three days later it disappeared completely. Now fast forward 15 years later, my right hand is shaking again."

Stress is a very important factor that influences when and to what degree your symptoms will surface (you will learn more about the impact of stress in later chapters). This is an important observation and in part the premise for this book's message…you have an important role to play in how your symptoms present and change over time.

Parkinson's disease should not be understood and analyzed as simply a brain disease. Your actions, experience and environment can influence your symptoms!

Making the Diagnosis

For most people, PD is a clinical diagnosis based not on blood tests or brain scans; but on medical history, description of symptoms and clinical examination. In this modern day world filled with data, medical tests and diagnostic procedures, the fact that diagnosis depends on the exchange that ocurrs in the examination room is surprising and in some situations leads the patient to question the diagnosis. So what is the criteria for diagnosis?

The clinical diagnosis of PD requires the presence of two out of three primary movement symptoms: tremor, rigidity (stiffness) notably in the arms or legs and bradykinesia (slowness.) Symptom onset is gradual and asymmetric (present on one side of the body.) A complete neurologic examination is important as certain clues on examination will point to other diagnoses such as stroke or multiple sclerosis.

The DaTSCAN[1] was approved for use in 2012 and can help differentiate PD tremor from another type of tremor such as essential or familial tremor. DaTSCAN is a nuclear medicine scan that indirectly measures dopamine nerve cells in the basal ganglia, an area of the brain affected in PD. It is important to note that this test cannot differentiate PD from other types of parkinsonism so is it helpful only in very specific situations. The picture below compares the DaTSCAN image of a person without PD (left) to early, mid and late stage PD. The center of each image shows the concentration of dopamine nerve cells and illustrates how one side is less affected (less symptoms).

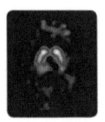  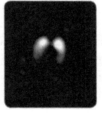 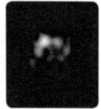

As previously noted, non-motor symptoms may occur before motor symptoms and their presence can help support diagnosis. Researchers are actively studying this pre-clinical syndrome with the hope of diagnosing PD earlier and more accurately. Earlier diagnosis will become increasingly important as scientists develop therapies that are neuroprotective, that is, treatments that slow disease

---

[1] Image courtesy of GE Healthcare

progression. You will learn more about neuroprotection in the Neuroplasticity chapter.

Blood tests are not routinely needed for diagnosis but can be helpful to insure an alternative diagnosis does not exist when atypical or uncommon findings on examination or history are noted. These tests are listed on the next page.

Specific examination clues usually exist to differentiate PD from other conditions. In most cases, laboratory tests are not needed. When the diagnosis is uncertain, the PD specialist may want to monitor the person every 6 months to avoid giving an incorrect diagnosis and unnecessary medication.

Common Tests to Identify Conditions that Mimic PD

Blood or Urine Tests	Imaging	Other	Common reason(s) test is performed
Thyroid tests			Low thyroid function can cause fatigue, muscle pain, constipation, depression. High thyroid function can cause tremor.
Vitamin B12			Low levels can cause fatigue, balance problems and cognitive changes
Copper & Ceruloplasmin			Wilson's disease- a hereditary condition associated with psychiatric and Parkinson like motor symptoms
	Brain or MRI		Stroke sometimes called vascular parkinsonism and Normal Pressure Hydrocephalus
	DaTSCAN		Differentiates parkinsonian syndromes from Essential tremor
	MRI or CT Scan	Lumbar Puncture	Spinal tap combined with imaging to confirm Normal Pressure Hydrocephalus (early walking, bladder and thinking problems)
		EMG	Electrical muscle testing to assess for certain diseases of nerve and muscle that cause weakness, early speech, and swallowing problems
		Cognitive Screen	Testing usually performed by a Neuropsychologist. Helpful when early cognitive problems are present suggesting dementia or psychological causes.

Other Parkinson-like Syndromes

Many conditions have similar symptoms of bradykinesia, rigidity or tremor but are differentiated from PD by the following:

- Symmetric symptoms (symptoms begin on both sides of body)
- Rigidity in the neck and trunk at onset instead of arms and legs
- Early balance, speech or swallowing problems
- Early and significant cognitive problems
- Early and significant *autonomic* dysfunction (dizziness or fainting, bladder control problems, sexual dysfunction)
- Muscle loss or muscle weakness
- Change in vision due to eye movement problems especially with upward gaze

Examples of parkinson-like syndromes (sometimes called atypical parkinsonism) include multiple system atrophy (early balance and autonomic dysfunction), progressive supranuclear palsy (early cognitive, balance and eye movement problems), Lewy body disease (Parkinson like symptoms, cognitive problems and hallucinations within the first year of diagnosis), and normal pressure hydrocephalus (slow, 'sticky' walking along with cognitive problems and bladder incontinence). Parkinson like symptoms can also be caused by medicines such as neuroleptics (antipsychotic medicines used for psychosis and sometimes depression) and some anti-nausea medicines.

How are Parkinson's symptoms measured?

The Hoehn & Yahr and Unified Parkinson's Disease Rating Scale (UPDRS) are two rating scales used to measure severity of movement and activities of daily living. These scales may not always reflect how you feel in early stages since they are somewhat subjective and reflect a brief period of time. Often the most important information obtained during your medical appointment is obtained by 'telling your story' of how your symptoms or diagnosis impacts your day, night, activities, emotions, family and coping. Be sure to focus on more than just your outward physical symptoms and spend a few minutes in the appointment talking about these issues that are important to your wellbeing between your medical appointments.

Modified Hoehn & Yahr Scale

Stage	Symptoms	Average Time of Progression to Next Stage
1	Unilateral (one side of body), Minimal problems	
1.5	Unilateral and Axial (middle of body)	
2	Bilateral (both sides of body) or Axial without balance problems	**20 months**
2.5	Bilateral with mild postural instability (easily recovers)	**62 months**
3	Bilateral disease: mild to moderate disability with impaired postural reflexes; physically independent	**25 months**
4	Severely disabling disease; still able to walk or stand but with assistance	**24 months**
5	Wheelchair or bed bound	**26 months**

Note: This scale was first published by Drs. Hoehn and Yahr and later modified to include stages 1.5 and 2.5. Time of progression described above was reported by in a study by Dr. Zhao (see reference section.)

Predicting the Future

Managing change and uncertainty is difficult and sometimes a source of concern or fear early in disease. *"What can I expect over the next 2, 5 or 10 Years?"* This is one of the most common questions asked during appointments. There is no 'crystal ball' to predict the future but there are general trends or patterns of change that are expected. The prior table lists average times to progression from one stage to the next as measured in a study of 695 people already living with PD. This information, although helpful, may not apply to you. **Why?**

Because you are taking the steps toward better management, prevention and emotional wellbeing that will impact how you feel today and how things change in the future.

For instance, after reviewing the movement and mobility changes described in each stage on the prior page, you will understand the benefit of beginning an exercise or therapy program <u>today</u> with the following focus:

- Coordination and use of both sides of the body
- Balance
- Axial motor control- posture, back and spine flexibility, strength, and speech
- Power and endurance

Learning more about these important steps and lifestyle changes can give you a sense of control and is a powerful first step toward combating the fear of change and uncertainty.

How did I get Parkinson's disease?

Familial or genetic PD (parent, sibling or child also with PD) accounts for only 15% of PD. Not all genes associated with PD have been discovered, but familial cases are most commonly associated with these genetic mutations: *LRRK2, PARK2, PARK7, PINK1,* or *SNCA.* Most cases of PD, however, are sporadic; likely resulting from a complex interaction between environment and genetics.

Research suggests that genetics is more likely to play a role in people with symptom onset prior to age 40 yrs. A recent study found that 16% of people with young onset PD have abnormal genes with the most common being Parkin, LRRK2 and glucocerebrosidase.

Having one family member with PD does not always increase the risk of developing PD. The cumulative lifetime risk of developing PD for a first degree family member (parent, sibling or child) in the US is between 3% and 7%. This is compared to a lifetime risk of developing PD of 1 to 2% in the general population.

Genetics do not tell the whole story. Some genes, such as alpha synuclein, are thought to cause PD and some such as the more common genes, *GBA* and LRKK2 are associated with or simply modify the risk of developing PD. Genetic testing is available but is not routinely obtained as the actual significance of an abnormal gene is still unknown. The most common genes identified to date increase the risk but do not cause the disease.

Commercial companies offer very limited genetic testing of saliva for a specific PD gene and partner with research organizations to collect and analyze genetic information from a large number of people. This could help advance the science of genetics and PD. These companies do not offer a full spectrum of genetic testing or counseling and should not be used to confirm or rule out a diagnosis. Genetic counseling is available in many large medical centers and university programs and is an important step in understanding the complexity of genetic testing for you and the family, influence on insurance qualification and other unforeseen issues.

Nature v. Nurture

Both nature and nurture play a role as a combination of genetics and environment work together to increase a person's risk of developing PD. In the majority of cases, genetic abnormalities do not actually cause the disease but instead increases susceptibility or risk of developing PD. In addition, there is a long list of potential environmental or lifetime activities that may increase the risk for developing PD. Although these factors alone increase risk by a small amount they can have a cumulative effect. It is likely that multiple causes such as a combination of factors and/or genetic abnormalities work together to cause PD. This is called the *multiple hit hypotheses*. It is also important to understand that these conclusions are drawn from observations and statistical analysis of probability for large groups of people (epidemiologic or population studies) making it difficult to apply this information to you as a single individual.

Some of the factors that may increase the risk of developing PD:
- Advancing age
- Male gender
- Declining estrogen levels
- Family history of first degree relative with PD
- Head injury
- Rural living and drinking well water
- Pesticide exposure
- Industrial solvent exposure such as found in certain industries such as older dry cleaning techniques
- Low vitamin D level

There are also some factors that may protect or reduce the risk of developing PD. Whether focusing on some of these factors will slow down the changes after the diagnosis of PD is not yet known.
- Female gender
- Smoking (not recommended!)
- Exercise
- Coffee and green tea
- Diet high in vitamin B6 (bell peppers, spinach, unskinned baked potatoes, peas, yams, broccoli, asparagus, turnip greens, peanuts, cashews, hazelnuts, chick peas, lentils, soybeans)
- Peppers, berries

It is clear that the above list of environmental and lifestyle factors do influence the risk of developing PD. What is not known is whether these same factors influence disease progression once PD is diagnosed. What this information means to you, however, is very clear:

- Multiple factors can cause the PD.

- The scientific rationale or explanation for why certain factors cause PD is becoming clearer as is their role in health.

- Some of these factors are under our control or influence, enhance health and are therefore a worthy focus of attention.

- It is never too late to make healthy lifestyle choices.

PARKINSON'S DISEASE FACTS & MYTHS

Myth: Tremor must be present to be diagnosed with PD. Fact: About 20-30% of people with PD do not have tremor.

Myth: The DaTSCAN can diagnose PD. Fact: This scan can differentiate parkinsonian conditions from Essential tremor but cannot differentiate PD with other forms of parkinsonism.

Myth: I will need a wheelchair in 5 years. Fact: Each person's disease, health and symptoms are different and progression is influenced by treatment, general health and lifestyle.

Myth: There is nothing I can do that will make a difference. Fact: Life choices will influence your future with PD.

Alter Your Course

1. Scientific evidence proves PD is caused by a combination of genetics and environment. You, your lifestyle and the environment you live in can make a difference. Learn what is within your power to make a positive difference.

2. Parkinson's is a progressive condition. Although each person's condition is different, there are similarities in how symptoms progress. Use your knowledge of how symptoms typically progress and put a plan in place to combat these problems, i.e. target speech, motor coordination, balance, endurance, stress, depression and cognition.

MOVEMENT &
NEUROPERFORMANCE
CENTER

COPING WITH THE DIAGNOSIS

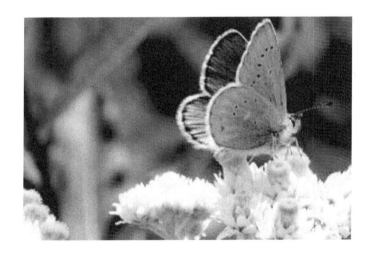

'Change can yield unexpected results.'

Photo by Sierra Farris

Reaction to Diagnosis

There are stages of adjustment or coping that one goes through after diagnosis just as there are stages of Parkinson's disease. These stages are often similar to the stages of grief defined by Dr. Kubler-Ross.

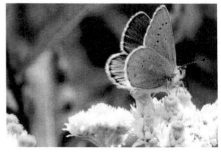

As a recently diagnosed person, you may have experienced one or more of these stages, reflecting different levels of adjustment, adaptation and readiness to deal with the disease. Not everyone experiences each stage nor do people progress from one stage to the next in a linear fashion.

- Denial. *"This isn't happening to me."*
- Anger. *"I don't deserve this."*
- Fear. *"I am worried about how this changes things."*
- Depression or Setbacks. *"My future is doomed."*
- Acceptance and Adaptation. *"I will deal with this and move on."*

Although your experience after diagnosis is more complex than these simple stages, the change from one stage to the next suggest a modifiable and dynamic experience when living with a chronic condition. Just as Parkinson's can bring change that will impact your life, so will your <u>reaction</u> to the diagnosis impact your life. The important thing to note is that you have, to some degree, a choice as to how you respond and change over time.

Take a moment to review the following chart highlighting each reactionary stage. An example of different reactions to diagnosis is listed for each stage. Coupled with each reaction is an alternative response designed to increase resiliency and ability to cope no matter what stage you are facing.

A counselor and psychologist can help you and your family work through the emotions you are feeling about diagnosis. This is true even if you feel you are coping fairly well as these professionals can help you better handle any changes the future may bring.

Emotional Stages Associated with Diagnosis

Stage	Reaction	Response
Denial	I'll ignore my symptoms and they will go away.	I'll seek help from my doctor and others.
Anger	This is not fair, why did it happen to me?	I'll try and focus on what I have and not just what I may lose.
Fear	I am so worried about my future.	I am worried but I'll optimize each moment, live for today and make plans for the future so that I am in control.
Setbacks	I'm getting worse, it's hopeless.	I'll work on the things that I know I can improve and find ways to adjust to the things I cannot.
Acceptance	I have a disease and will never get better.	I can get better with treatment and lifestyle choices I can control. With support I will adjust and adapt to the ups and downs that come with this condition.

Do you recognize these reactions? The table highlights two over riding themes:

1. *Reaction v. Response.* A reaction to a problem is a quick action or feeling that we engage automatically without thought. A response is a thoughtful and intentional action or feeling that we chose based on the outcome we desire.

2. *Negative v. Positive.* Some responses lead to a more comfortable acceptance while others may make it difficult to move in a forward and positive direction.

Simply being aware that these reactions are normal and that you have a choice in how you respond within each stage can help you move towards positive acceptance.

Hope

Hope has many sources. Hope grows from the strength gained through support from others, your spiritual beliefs and personal values that shine forth during difficult times. Hope also blossoms with the understanding that you can influence your future. The awareness that you have a choice in your attitude after diagnosis and that you can impact your disease with positive lifestyle choices will sustain the lifeline of hope.

Alter Your Course

1. Scientific evidence proves PD is caused by a combination of genetics and environment. You, your lifestyle and the environment you live in can make a difference. Learn what is in your power to make a positive difference.

2. Parkinson's is a progressive condition. Although each person's condition is different, there are similarities in how symptoms progress. Use your knowledge of how symptoms typically progress and put a plan in place to combat these problems, i.e. target speech, motor coordination, balance, endurance, depression and cognition.

3. **Be aware of how your reaction to the diagnosis impacts your activities and attitude. Recognize that you have a choice in how you respond and this choice can include the decision to focus on the positive steps you can take rather than getting stuck in a negative reaction to what you have lost. You control the path you choose.**

LIFE'S JOURNEY
SETTING YOUR COURSE

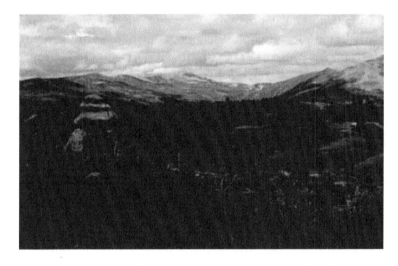

Courage, knowledge and intention will guide the way

Photo by Sierra Farris

Parkinson's disease is an unexpected, and unwanted, twist and turn in your life journey. Like any journey there is uncertainty about what lies ahead, how things will change or where your life with PD will take you. Although you cannot 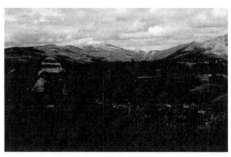 completely control your future, certain choices you make can guide your course in the best direction.

Change is an opportunity to refocus your priorities. No one can predict their future but they can lay the foundation for their future to unfold in a particular direction. Like any journey, the first step is to set your intentions and take deliberate steps toward positive action. Your diagnosis presents you with this opportunity- to take action and choose how you will move forward.

This chapter is one example in how to prepare for the unexpected. The information described here is explored in further detail throughout the remainder of this book.

Get the Facts- How Much and When

Learn about PD symptoms and how they change over time. Understand available medical and non-medical treatments. Education builds confidence and provides the tools you will need to play an active part in your care. You may need to advocate for therapies that prevent or delay physical changes. Ultimately, education will give you some control over the disease. Remember that everyone will be different in their approach and how they utilize information. Some people thrive by learning all they can, including the good and the bad. Yet others, especially in early stages may find that too much information causes unnecessary anxiety about the future.

Think about which approach works best for you before you dive into learning about PD *full steam ahead.* Do you need to pace yourself? The internet is full of information, some of it good, some of it not. Be sure to seek credible sources by respected professionals and foundations. Look for information that is designed to empower, inspire and offer practical guidance rather than read like an encyclopedia of facts. If too much information is overwhelming then you may want to start with your doctor and allow some time to adjust after the diagnosis before learning more.

Family, Friends & Support

Your first few years with PD will be less scary and isolating if you reach out to others. It is comforting to have others for support, guidance and to lean on when needed. Talk with family and friends about what is happening. Seek the advice of others who have *'been in your shoes'* and have found ways to cope.

A support group is one way to meet others who can help. Each support group has its own *'personality'*, focus and style. If you are not sure if you are ready for a support group, start by asking the leader how many attendees are recently diagnosed and in your age group to gauge whether the group is the right fit for you. You may also find it helpful to talk with the support group leader about group dynamics; for instance does the group focus on guest speakers and lecture? If so, you can pick and choose which day to attend. Be wary of groups that focus entirely on the negative without time for support, a motivational message and/or positive solutions.

Take Charge of Your Medical Care

Parkinson's is a life-long condition. As such, your symptoms will change and treatments will be modified to respond to these changes. New advances in our (your) understanding of disease and what you as an individual can do for your wellbeing means that you will have many different options and strategies for your care. Your personal healthcare values and preferences add even more options for care that is tailored to you as a person and not just the symptoms of disease.

As one patient stated when describing her healthcare, *"I feel best when I am part of the (treatment) solution."*

Be a part of your solution.

Partner with your medical team to help them make the best choices for you. Do this by preparing for your medical visits, setting goals and objectives, keeping notes when necessary, organizing your information and healthcare data in one place and advocating for the care you need. This important topic is reviewed in more detail in the next chapter.

Lifestyle

You are not your disease. You are a person living with PD. Although this is an obvious statement, it is also a very important reminder. Often we place our focus of attention on the tangible features of disease, symptoms, and their physiologic and neurochemical causes. Yet our neurochemical and physiologic changes occur within a broader network of cellular interactions and neural interconnections responding to our body as a system, the environment we live in and our personal life experiences.

Neuroplasticity is a term used to define changes in brain activity in response to our activities and experiences. In other words, your lifestyle not only changes your physical health but also your brain function. Certain lifestyle activities may even change how PD progresses, a term called neuroprotection. Create your brain enhancing lifestyle through:

- Therapeutic Exercise
- Optimal Nutrition
- Stress Management
- Positive experiences & Attitude
- Creative, Challenging and Meaningful actions

Priorities

Life changing events like PD, do offer the opportunity to set priorities in how you live your life. Appreciating the small moments help stay focused on the positives. Prioritizing what is positive and meaningful is an important step in charting your new course.

Attitude and Gratitude

It is easy to get caught up in regrets, bitterness and anger about what PD has 'taken' from you. Counter this with acts of kindness- to yourself and others. Find something each day for which you are grateful. Over time you will train your brain to let the positive thoughts overrule the negative.

Spirituality and Compassion

A full life does not depend on how graceful you are, how fast you move, how long you can walk or how physically strong you are. A full life is one filled with personal meaning, sense of value and compassion. *What adds meaning, value and passion to your life? Do you have a spiritual connection, relationship to humanity or nature that desires cultivation?* Do not let Parkinson's take this from you.

Life Planning

Feeling unsettled is common when the future is uncertain. Having a plan for change will help you remain in control. Learn about the roles of a healthcare proxy, living will and power of attorney. Investigate services that are available in your community and long-term care opportunities in the event you are in need. Discuss and write down your healthcare wishes at end of life so that these wishes are respected. This topic will be covered in greater detail in the Family, Relationships & Work chapter.

Alter Your Course

1. Scientific evidence proves PD is caused by a combination of genetics and environment. You, your lifestyle and the environment you live in can make a difference. Learn what is within your power to make a positive difference.

2. Parkinson's is a progressive condition. Although each person's condition is different, there are similarities in how symptoms progress. Use your knowledge of how symptoms typically progress and put a plan in place to combat these problems, i.e. target speech, motor coordination, balance, endurance, stress, depression and cognition.

3. Be aware of how your reaction to the diagnosis impacts your activities and attitude. Recognize that you have a choice in how you respond and this choice can include the decision to focus on the positive steps you can take rather than getting stuck in a negative reaction to what you have lost. You control the path you choose.

4. **Plan your journey with attention to knowledge, support, medical care, lifestyle, attitude and compassion.**

HOPE & RESILIENCY

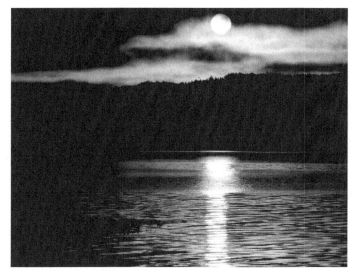

"Not my sunset but my sunrise"

-Photo courtesy of Nathan Henwood, Thriving with PD

"You can't change that you have Parkinson's disease but you can change how you choose to live with PD."

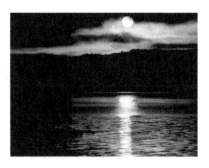

Many people with PD understand that how one chooses to live with PD is key to personal wellbeing.

Each chapter in this book is filled with ways you can make a difference and set the stage for a bettter future with PD. In this chapter we will review the personal behaviors and ideas that set the foundation for a strong future.

Power of Diagnosis

Often symptoms are present for months or even years before diagnosis. Young individuals or those without tremor may be misdiagnosed or experience a delay in the diagnosis. Symptoms may not be present all the time or confused with getting older. The fluctuating nature of PD increases focus and worry about symptoms and what it all means.

The words *"you have Parkinson's disease"* can come with a flood of emotions. Whether you know someone with PD, have seen people with PD on TV or in your doctor's office; your imagination can drift to the worst possible scenario. Your mind may paint a picture of what PD 'looks' like, but you are not that person. You have the power to influence the disease and how you cope, adapt, and respond to changes. As Janice from *Advice in the Trenches* reminds us:

"You can identify with the disease and focus on your symptoms, fearing future symptoms even before they occur. This might even make symptoms happen earlier.
OR
You can use your diagnosis as a spring board for positive lifestyle and personal change."

Diagnosis can bring relief. Relief not because you want PD but because the diagnosis validates the problems you are having and gives you the motivation to take action.

"I knew something was wrong. I saw a lot of doctors for muscle pain before finally getting my diagnosis. Before diagnosis, I felt like I was not taken seriously and I didn't know what to do. Although my diagnosis of PD was a shock, I felt like OK, now I can do something about it. I took steps to learn about PD and what I could rather than passively sit on the side lines and watch my symptoms get worse. Simply knowing gave me a sense of control."

Balance

Maintaining balance in life and your views of treatment is important after diagnosis. Everyone is different in how they deal with adversity, ranging from the extreme to the balanced. Some people use denial and ignore symptoms or the diagnosis. Although denial is helpful when you are otherwise feeling overwhelmed, it does mean that you are less likely to focus on positive attitude, lifestyle and treatments important for your condition. The stress and reaction to the diagnosis can become buried under the surface. The other end of the spectrum is the person that focuses so much on their disease and treatment that even positive change can have negative consequences. Any resemblance to life 'normalcy' is lost; personal identity becomes the disease, and search for the ideal treatment becomes life's new focus. Although this approach is more proactive, the focus on disease can cause undue stress and negative consequences on the person and family.

A balanced approach means learning and taking steps towards better health, but at the same time recognizing that you are not your PD and life continues to exist without PD. With this in mind, you can fight the disease but not become the disease.

"When I was first diagnosed my whole life was focused around PD. Constantly reading about the disease. Am I exercising enough? Eating the right things? Constantly pursuing new treatments- I became my disease. Never satisfied and always worried that I was not doing enough...Now I approach my life with

PD on a much kinder note. I still eat well and exercise but don't beat myself up if I skip a day. I try not to lose myself to PD."

4 Ps- Preparation, Priority, Possibility and Positivity

Preparation. The first step toward being prepared is to learn about PD, symptoms, potential changes and treatment options. Learning about changes that typically occur over time can be stressful in the early stage. You may be experiencing only mild symptoms and may find it stressful to read about other problems that can occur over time. It is important to remember that everyone is different and that certainly applies to PD as well. You may never experience some of the symptoms you learn about and if you do, the goal is to reduce or prevent problems. By taking a proactive approach you can prevent or lessen symptoms rather than waiting for problems to occur and avoid being paralyzed by fear of the unknown. You will use the information you learn in the early stage for the following:

- Partner with your healthcare provider to optimize your therapy.
- Recognize treatment associated side effects.
- Establish a preventative therapy program to target potential future problems.
- Learn about other healthcare and healing professionals that can help.
- Be prepared if and when changes do occur.

Priority. Any life changing event brings with it the opportunity to take inventory of your life and renew or re-establish what truly is important to you and your family. Parkinson's disease does not define you but does affect how you see your life. With this new 'lens', you may see more clearly what is truly important giving you renewed focus and attention on these areas. This is common after diagnosis, and indeed throughout your journey with PD.

- Set realistic goals for yourself.
- Put a plan in place to reach those goals

"Parkinson's disease is the best thing that ever happened to me. Before (PD), all I cared about was my job and money. Now I pay more attention to my family. This makes me richer."

Possibility. The photograph introducing this chapter was taken by a person living well with PD. When I (Dr. Giroux) first saw this photo I commented on the beauty of the sunset. His response was inspiring:

"This is not the sunset but the sunrise. I feel that is what PD has given me. A chance to look at life anew, focusing on what is important to me. Without PD, I would be going through life without giving it any additional thought. With PD, I shape how (where) my life will go." Nathan PD for 11 years

- Seize the day. Create your *bucket list*.

Positivity. How we perceive our situation, our thoughts, feelings and attitude will impact how we feel, the life choices we make and even our response to treatment. The placebo effect is an example of how our thoughts impact what happens. The placebo effect increases along with the expectations we have for improvement and how valuable we perceive the treatment. In other words, if you expect a treatment or lifestyle change to make a positive difference there is a greater chance that it will.

With the power of positivity comes a broader and more expansive way of looking at and solving problems; leading to a broader array of solutions and ways of overcoming obstacles. Negative thoughts, on the other hand narrow our thoughts and minimize creative problem solving.

Mindfulness

Mindfulness is described as bringing your awareness to the moment with intention and without judgment. Mindfulness joins your mind, emotions, senses and body together as a whole. Bringing awareness to the moment helps you 'see' the moment. Non-judgment refers to the ability to simply notice a symptom, feeling, sensation or an experience without attaching a label or reaction. This practice can help you deal with moments that would otherwise bring distress. For instance, you may have negative thoughts about your tremor. The more you attach these thoughts to your tremor, the greater your negative reaction to tremor during moments you notice tremor. This distress creates then more tremor. The result is an escalating *snowball effect*.

We often spend too much time judging or mourning the past or worrying about the future that we are not present and fully appreciative of the present. This observation is especially important when living with a chronic condition and mindfulness is a helpful way to manage your worries about the future, uncertainty and feelings of losing control after diagnosis. We can control how we respond to our problems in the present and this will exert some control and impact on the future.

Mindfulness also helps bring your attention to life's simple pleasures. When was the last time you saw the sunset with full attention, noticed the delicate nature of tiny dew drops, a smile or friendly gesture from another person? Mindfulness can be a formal practice such as meditation, or an informal practice bringing moments of mindfulness into your day.

Connection

Mindfulness connects our thoughts, emotions and sensations to the moment. Positivity opens us up to life's possibilities even in times of stress. Setting priorities help guide life choices toward that which is meaningful for you.

Meaning, value and purpose are an important part of your existence. This does not lessen with the diagnosis of Parkinson's and as Nathan reminds us with his beautiful picture of the sunrise that life can even be enriched with PD.

Our spirit lies at the very core of who we are, what we cherish and hold true, how we act and what we do.

"How often do you hear (or read) the terms healing, spirituality and Parkinson's in the same sentence or together in conversation. Our discussion of Parkinson's care usually focuses on the physical body and its treatment. Yet healing and spirituality is of critical importance in any illness but especially PD since it broadens one's definition of self and care beyond the physical body. Our spiritual self can remain strong, grow stronger and heal at all stages of PD."

– Monique Giroux MD

Spirituality is personal, goes beyond organized religion and has different meanings for different people. Spirituality includes:

- *How we think-* Questions about meaning, what is important or what gives purpose to your life. As a person with Parkinson's you may find yourself asking the question-*how do I continue along my life's path? do I start over and change my life path?*

- *How we feel-* This includes feelings or emotions such as love, connection, community, hope, inner peace, joy, sorrow, desire, empathy, acceptance, and forgiveness. How we feel about life can change after a diagnosis such as Parkinson's bringing clarity to a higher purpose.

- *How we act-* This encompasses our relationships with others, commitment to church or organization, prayer and meditation, generosity in giving and support, and the very act of caring for ourselves and others. After the diagnosis, a new world can open up that may include new relationships, goals, adventures and connections.

The simple act of meeting over a cup of coffee, joining a support group or attending a community meeting is more than just a social or educational event. These encounters are opportunities that allow you to share your life with others living with PD, offer what you have learned and give you the opportunity to reach out and connect and in that moment together make a difference.

"I have met so many great people since my diagnosis. People I would have never met otherwise. It is a community. The support, encouragement, and compassion I get and give is priceless. Sometimes I see this as a gift."

Alter Your Course

1. Scientific evidence proves PD is caused by a combination of genetics and environment. You, your lifestyle and the environment you live in can make a difference. Learn what is within your power to make a difference.

2. Parkinson's is a progressive condition. Although each person's condition is different, there are similarities in how symptoms progress. Use your knowledge of symptoms associated with disease progression and put a plan in place to combat these problems, i.e. speech, motor coordination, balance, endurance, stress, depression and cognition.

3. Be aware of how your reaction to diagnosis impacts your activities and attitude. Recognize that you have a choice in how you respond and this choice can include the decision to focus on the positive steps you can take rather than the negative.

4. Change the direction of your journey with attention to these steps- knowledge, support, medical care, lifestyle, attitude and compassion. You control the path you choose.

5. **Parkinson's can be an opportunity. An opportunity to reset life's priorities and balance, experience life's richness in the moment, focus on the positive, what is possible and what adds true meaning to your life.**

MOVEMENT &
NEUROPERFORMANCE
CENTER

NAVIGATING YOUR HEALTHCARE

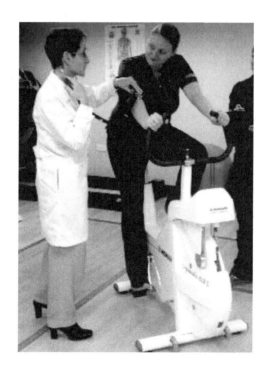

It takes a team.

Finding The Right Doctor

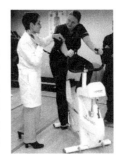

This may be the first time you have been faced with a serious or chronic illness. You may have had little need to see a physician let alone a specialist. Or perhaps PD is one of many medical conditions you are living with each requiring specific treatments, multiple healthcare providers and frequent check-ups.

Whatever your healthcare experience, finding a doctor that has expertise in PD is a good first step for anyone recently diagnosed. Consider seeing a neurologist with a focus on PD with additional training (called a fellowship) in movement disorders. However, some general neurologists may have many patients with PD and may be very experienced in movement disorder's care.

Since PD is a life-long condition, you will do best with a physician or healthcare provider that you can develop a trusting and therapeutic relationship. Communication is an important part of your care and having a provider that listens to how you feel will enhance your care and adjustment to the diagnosis. Communication is so important that a study of factors that affect quality of life in PD showed a strong correlation between the quality of communication between provider and patient and perceived impact on quality of life.

"My doctor watched me walk, talked to me for 5 minutes, then said I had Parkinson's disease, wrote a prescription and left. I was in shock I didn't know what it all meant."

Walking out of the appointment with a prescription having no idea what the doctor said, what treatment is recommended or why, can leave you feeling more confused and powerless than when you walked in. Don't let this happen to you. Be an active participant in your care and treatment decisions.

The right doctor or healthcare provider will be the person that listens and makes the effort to understand your situation, your values and treatment preferences. This includes describing treatment options in terms you can understand, and involves you and your family in treatment decisions.

46

The following checklist can help you choose the find the medical provider that is the best fir for you:

- Does your healthcare provider have training, expertise and/or interest in treating PD?
- Does your healthcare provider listen to you?
- Does your healthcare provider spend the time needed to treat you?
- Does your healthcare provider ask your opinion or care preference?
- Is your healthcare provider open to new ways of doing or thinking about you and your condition?
- Does your healthcare provider explain why treatments are being suggested or used?
- Do you leave the office in full understanding about what to do and why?
- Does your healthcare provider include your partner, spouse or other important people in your life in the appointments and discussion?
- Does your healthcare provider take a proactive and preventative approach to your care?
- Is your healthcare provider only interested in medicines, research or surgery; or do they also embrace a holistic approach?
- Does your healthcare provider refer to rehabilitation therapists?

Assemble Your Team

The next step is to be sure that you have the right team members on your *'medical team'* based on your needs and philosophical beliefs about health and healing (learn more about this in the complementary therapy chapter). This may include but certainly not limited to physicians, physician assistants, nurses, counselors, rehabilitation specialists, alternative medicine therapists and healing arts specialists.

Don't forget to include your primary care physician or general health practitioner. Many people with PD focus so much on their disease that they forget about their general health. Use this as an opportunity to educate and update your primary doctor on the latest therapies.

- Do not wait until you have a problem to see your primary doctor. Follow through with a yearly examination even if you are not ill so he/she can understand your healthcare needs and can focus on health and prevention.

- Remember that your PD symptoms are influenced by your general health.

Look to more than doctors to round out your care. Your neurologist may work closely with physician assistants and nurses. These individuals often have a different perspective and an approach that can complement your care.

Rehabilitation specialist, counselors and healing arts specialists are also important team members as outlined in the following chapters.

Navigating Your Medical Care

Most metropolitan areas have PD experts available but some communities have limited PD resources. Many people that live in rural areas travel to a PD specialist periodically to stay current on treatment options and to learn about the latest research. If you cannot travel to a specialty center, an option would be to have your local support group organize an educational event and invite a PD expert to speak about the latest treatment and research findings for PD. There are also a growing number of local and regional PD foundations that now focus on education with great online resources.

Holistic Brain Health offers treatment and lifestyle support at www.drgiroux.com.

Personalizing Your Care

Although some people think that treating newly diagnosed PD is much simpler than treating someone with moderate to advanced PD, this is not the case. Each person is different in respect to their disease, lifestyle, emotional adjustment, coping, level of support and treatment goals.

Care must be tailored to you not just the disease.

Not everyone will decide to begin medicine right away. You may be interested in natural therapies, exercise, diet or other alternative therapies. You may need counseling or more support to feel well. You will feel empowered if you take charge of your health and your commitment will serve to reinforce treatment and lifestyle changes. Be sure to:

- Set goals for your appointments.
- Prioritize your symptoms and goals.
- Decide who will be involved in your therapy and treatment.
- Talk to your team about your concerns, ideas and interests in medication, research trials, and non-medical therapies.
- Be honest with your team about what you can (will) and cannot (will not) do.

Be Prepared

There are a few steps that you can take to get the most out of your medical care. Being prepared for your medical visit is an important step in making sure your needs are met during your time with your medical provider. Bring someone with you to take notes and help you understand and remember what is being said during your appointment.

Simple steps to optimize your medical visit are:

- Take the time needed to carefully prepare for your appointments. This will help you get the most out of your appointments and insure that care is tailored to your individual needs.

- Obtain copies of your healthcare provider's questionnaire in advance so that you can complete it accurately. Don't assume your doctor already knows or remembers specific information about you.

- Have a goal for each appointment. Write that goal down and leave a space to record your answer or solution. This way you are sure to have a treatment plan in place by the end of the appointment.

- Write down your questions prior to your visit.

- Set priorities. Remember that your time with your provider is limited so use it wisely. Your healthcare provider may not be able to answer numerous questions but should be able to focus on your top priorities. Also ask questions in the beginning rather than waiting until the appointment is over to ask your questions.

- Keep a list of all medicines you are taking or have tried in the past. Record the dose, when you took it during the day and any positive effects or side effects. Remember PD is a lifelong condition and this information will be very helpful in the years to come when a change in medicine is needed.

- When you get a new prescription for a medication, record why you are taking it, what to expect, and the most common side effects.

- Learn your healthcare provider's policies on issues such as between office phone calls, prescription refills and form completion so you know how to get your needs met between appointments.

- Bring someone with you to help you stay focused, remember and understand what is being said during an appointment.

- Understand when and from whom you should seek help as your symptoms change. This may include other professionals such as counselors, social work, nutritionists, physical therapists, occupational therapists and speech therapists. The *Rehabilitation*

Worksheet located in the chapter on nonmedical therapies will help you understand how these specialists can help.

More Than Medicine

Living your best with PD may mean setting some new priorities for yourself or renewing your commitment to positive lifestyle change. As you will learn there is no single focus or 'magic bullet' but a holistic balance that is best- a balance that focuses on disease when needed and wellness when possible.

Alter Your Course

1. Scientific evidence proves PD is caused by a combination of genetics and environment. You, your lifestyle and the environment you live in can make a difference. Learn what is within your power to make a positive difference.

2. Parkinson's is a progressive condition. Although each person's condition is different, there are similarities in how symptoms progress. Use your knowledge of how symptoms typically progress and put a plan in place to combat these problems, i.e. target speech, motor coordination, balance, endurance, stress, depression and cognition.

3. Be aware of how your reaction to the diagnosis impacts your activities and attitude. Recognize that you have a choice in how you respond and this choice can include the decision to focus on the positive steps you can take rather than getting stuck in a negative reaction to what you have lost. You control the path you choose.

4. Plan your journey with attention to knowledge, support, medical care, lifestyle, attitude and compassion.

5. **Be an active member of your health care team and strive for the best results. Prepare for appointments, organize your healthcare data, set goals and assemble your team.**

MOVEMENT &
NEUROPERFORMANCE
CENTER

MEDICATION

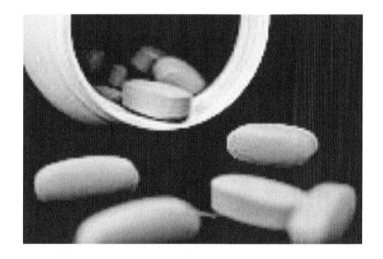

Medications are important for optimal brain health and motor control

As you have learned, Parkinson's disease is associated with a loss of dopamine producing nerve cells in the basal ganglia. Movement problems such as tremor, stiffness, slowness, and shuffling improve with medications that essentially 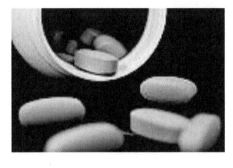 replace declining levels of dopamine. In some situations, nonmotor symptoms such as sleep, pain, mood and cognition also improve with dopaminergic medicines. PD medications and potential side effects are reviewed below.

Levodopa

Levodopa is one of the oldest medications used for PD and is still the most effective medicine for movement and has one of the lowest side effect profiles. Levodopa is absorbed in the small intestine, transported through the blood brain barrier and into the brain where it is absorbed by dopamine nerve cells. A chemical reaction occurs in the nerve cells converting levodopa to dopamine. Essentially, levodopa will restore inadequate levels of brain dopamine improving movement symptoms. Levodopa is combined with carbidopa (combination is called carbidopa/levodopa or trade Sinemet®, Parcopa®) Carbidopa prevents levodopa conversion to dopamine outside the brain both reducing nausea as a side effect and allowing more levodopa to enter the brain where it is needed. Carbidopa/levodopa is available in the following strengths:

- Regular: 10/100, 25/100 and 25/250
- Slow release formula: 25/100 and50/200
- Dissolvable formula: 25/100 and 25/250

(Note: 25/100 refers to 25mg carbidopa and 100mg levodopa).

Make sure you know which formulation you are taking as this is a major source of medication error.

MAOB Inhibitors

Monoamine oxidase type B (MAOB) inhibitors slow the breakdown of dopamine in the brain enhancing dopamine effectiveness. This class of medicines can be used as initial therapy in early stage.

- Selegiline (Eldepryl®, Zelopar®): 5mg once to twice daily, 1.25mg dissolvable tab one to two daily
- Rasagiline (Azilect®): 0.5mg and 1mg once daily

Amantadine

Amantadine (Symmetrel®) is a medication originally used to treat the flu but later found to improve PD motor symptoms. Amantadine can be used in early disease but is more commonly used to reduce dyskinesia, a problem experienced in later stages. Common dose range is 100mg one to three times a day. Amantadine can cause a lacy brown rash and swelling most often seen in the legs with long-term use. Other side effects are listed in the subsequent section. Amantadine is metabolized through the kidneys and people with kidney disease may require lower doses.

Dopamine Agonists

Dopamine agonists are a group of medications that mimic the effects of dopamine at neighboring nerve cells. These medications have a longer lasting affect and can help control symptoms over a longer period of the day. The following are dopamine agonists used in the USA.

- Ropinirole (Requip®)-
  - Immediate release- usually prescribed 3 times a day 0.25mg, 0.5mg, 1.0mg, 2mg, 3mg, 4mg, 5mg and 6mg
  - Extended Release (Requip XL®) - once day preparation 2mg, 4mg, 6mg, 8mg and 12mg
- Pramipexole (Mirapex®) –
  - Immediate release- usually prescribed 3 times day 0.125mg, 0.25mg, 0.5mg, 0.75mg, 1.0mg and 1.5mg

55

o Extended Release (Mirapex ER®) once day preparation 0.375mg, 0.75mg, 1.5mg, 2.25mg, 3mg, 3.75mg and 4.5mg

- Rotigotine Patch (Neupro®)- Once daily 2mg, 3mg, 4mg, 6mg, and 8mg patch

The following medications are used in moderate and advanced stages of Parkinson's disease and are not typically used in early disease.

COMT Inhibitors

Catechol-o-methyl-transferase (COMT) inhibitors block the metabolism or chemical degradation of levodopa in the body allowing the effect of levodopa to last longer. This group of medicines is used to treat end of dose wearing off associated with levodopa therapy in moderate disease and are not used in early disease. There are two COMT inhibitors:

- Entacapone (Comtan®, Stalevo®). Entacapone 200mg can be taken with carbidopa/levodopa. A combination pill called Stalevo® combines carbidopa/levodopa and entacapone into one pill. Stalevo is available in the following strengths:
    o 50mg, 75mg, 100mg, 125mg, 150mg and 200mg
- Tolcapone (Tasmar®) 100mg and 200mg is used less frequently due to potential liver toxicity requiring blood testing of liver function.
- Both of these medications can cause diarrhea.

Apomorphine (Apokyn®) is injected under the skin to provide very fast action typically within 20 minutes and is used for rescue treatment when wearing off is abrupt or unpredictable. This medicine is not used in early stages since wearing off is typically not a problem.

Side Effects

All dopaminergic medicines share similar side effects. These side effects are listed on the next page:

- Nausea and vomiting
- Heartburn
- Confusion (more common with agonists and amantadine)
- Hallucinations (more frequent with agonists and amantadine)
- Sedation, daytime sleepiness, sudden sleep attacks (may be more common with agonists)
- Impulsive or compulsive behaviors such as excessive gambling, overeating, hyper-sexuality problems (may be more common with agonists)
- Leg swelling (especially amantadine and agonists)
- Lightheadedness or dizziness (more common with agonists and amantadine)
- Insomnia (more common with selegiline)
- Constipation, memory loss, blurry vision, dry eyes, dry mouth and bladder retention (amantadine)

The decision to start medication and which medication to use is an individualized one based on symptom severity, side effect risks, activity or occupational needs, a person's philosophical views on medication and cost.

Some people feel an urgency to begin medicine immediately after diagnosis, wishing to greatly reduce or eliminate all symptoms. Others wish to 'put off medicines as long as possible.' Some people worry that medicines are *not natural, are toxic* or the effect will wear off and decide to focus on non-medical treatment such as exercise or supplements. A fear of medicine side effects and levodopa associated dyskinesia is also common (reviewed in the following pages.)

Beginning Medicine

Early and cautious use of medicine, however, can have positive benefits. Research investigating early use of the medicine rasagiline (Azilect®) showed that people who started this medicine earlier in disease did better than a comparative group that began therapy later. The reason for this finding is not clear. One proposed explanation is that rasagiline is neuroprotective, preventing vulnerable nerve cells from further damage. (Note: Although this is a possibility, research has not proven the assertion that rasagiline is neuroprotective.)

Alternatively, rasagiline may simply improve symptoms and change how you feel. As a result your lifestyle and wellbeing can improve for the better further enhancing positive change. Either way, these studies show that early use of medicine is not harmful and may in fact be beneficial when used wisely.

You will learn about the benefits of neuroplasticity in later chapters. Neuroplasticity describes a change in brain function influenced by activity and experiences. This concept may also apply to the timing of medicine. Medication can 'normalize' altered patterns of movement reinforcing positive brain changes that respond to enhanced motor fluidity, speed, precision and coordination. Conversely, waiting too long to start medicine can increase the impact of altered motor control due to PD and lead to compensatory changes in your motor system that ultimately impacts movement and brain function in a less positive direction. As activity levels drop off, your strength and endurance also fall off increasing fatigue levels and the need for assistance.

Medication dosage must be balanced to help movement but at a dosage that minimizes side effects.

Choosing the Right Medicine

There are multiple medicines for use in early disease including carbidopa/levodopa, dopamine agonists, amantadine and rasagiline. Which medicine is best for you depends on many factors including your age and side effect risk. The first medicine decision you and your healthcare provider will make is whether to begin levodopa or use a *levodopa conservative strategy.*

Levodopa Paradox

Levodopa is the most effective medicine for movement and has the lowest side effect profile. So why is this medicine so feared and misunderstood? Initially levodopa treats motor symptoms smoothly throughout the day. This changes with the emergence of *on-off* fluctuations as disease progresses and dopamine nerve cells degenerate. This first appears as a wearing off of medicine benefit before the next dose, a phenomenon called *end of dose wearing off*. Wearing off describes the return or worsening of symptoms prior to the next dose. Increase in medication strength, number of doses or use of additional medicines are then used to reduce off time. Dyskinesia (uncontrollable involuntary movements) can emerge as medications are increased or added. Levodopa has a greater risk of these problems due, in part, to the short half-life of levodopa in your bloodstream.

Longer acting medicines such as rasagiline and dopaminergic agonists when used alone have a low risk of dyskinesia. So the decision is simply to avoid levodopa…

Herein lies the paradox. Dopamine agonists have a higher risk of serious side effects such as confusion, hallucinations, dizziness, leg swelling and impulsivity control. These side effects limit the dose that is tolerated and even their use altogether in patients with higher risk of these problems. Rasagiline has a lower side effect risk but is often not strong enough to fully treat movement symptoms as the disease progresses. So treatment must be customized.

Levodopa may be the best first medicine when side effect risk is high such as older individuals, people on many medicines, with other significant medical problems affecting health or those with more severe movement problems. A levodopa conservative strategy can be used in younger people with less risk; beginning with agonists or rasagiline first and adding levodopa over the years when symptoms warrant. (In general, levodopa should be considered once significant walking, balance, speech and swallowing problems emerge.)

Talk to your healthcare provider about which medicine choice is best for you. Be sure to ask how side effect risk and long-term complications such as dyskinesia influence this choice.

Tremor and Dystonia

Tremor and dystonia can sometimes be difficult to treat even when medicine improves other symptoms. (Note: Dystonia is an excessive contraction of muscle causing pain, bending, twisting and posturing of the joints. This symptom is more common in people with young onset PD.) High doses of agonists and/or levodopa are sometimes required and with this a greater risk of side effects. The next chapter describes an effective treatment for tremor and dystonia, deep brain stimulation (DBS).

Clinical Research Trials- Are they right for you?

There are opportunities at diagnosis to participate in clinical research designed to measure the effect of early treatment and study the disease and/or treatment in individuals. There are many reasons to participate in research. One reason is the hope of finding a new treatment for you. Another is to contribute to future knowledge that will benefit others. Or perhaps you feel that clinical research is too risky, especially if a placebo may be involved.

Any new drug or new indication for an existing drug must go through a process governed by the federal Food and Drug Administration (FDA). The process involves many steps that may seem to take too long or cost too much. However, the FDA has the important task of protecting the public from unsafe or dangerous drugs. There are many research hurdles a potential drug must clear before being approved for use. Rigorous testing for safety and benefit in pre-clinical studies usually begins with animal or laboratory studies. Only drugs that pass the rigorous safety tests are made available for clinical trials involving people.

There are four phases of clinical trials. Phase I studies test the drug's safety and dosing requirements in a small number of people. Phase II helps to increase knowledge about side effects, dose and safety by including a larger number of people. Phase III extends phase II trials to include studies of efficacy in a larger group of people. The FDA will approve or disqualify a treatment based on phase III results. Phase IV studies continue to monitor treatment in the general population after a drug has been released for prescription use.

Many research trials include a placebo control. In such trials there is the chance you will not be given the active medicine but will instead receive an inactive pill or treatment. In "double blind" studies, neither the researcher nor the volunteer knows whether or not the active pill or treatment has been administered. A strong "placebo effect" is well-documented in Parkinson's studies. Simply expecting that a medicine or treatment will help can increase the chance of experiencing an improvement. Placebo-controlled trials, then, help insure that any benefits experienced are the result of the medication or treatment being tested, rather than the influence of positive expectations. Many placebo-controlled clinical trials are followed by an extension trial that allows all patients receiving placebo to receive the active drug.

All research is voluntary and participation is a personal decision that is protected by the law. There is always some form of personal cost involved when participating in a clinical research trial and participation should not be taken lightly. There should never be coercion, manipulation or judgment involved when a person is deciding whether or not to participate in research.

Clinical trials may narrow their study population by eliminating people that have certain medical problems, age ranges or disease duration. Although exclusionary criteria are important, the safety and effectiveness of a study medication in the general population may not be fully apparent until the drug is routinely prescribed to people with various other medical conditions in the population.

You must provide informed consent before you are allowed to participate in a clinical trial. The informed consent includes a document that defines the purpose of the research and its potential benefits and risks. Research trials and the informed consent must include the following principles:

- *Principle of respect for individuals.* That is, everyone has the right to information and the freedom to decide their treatment. In research, this is insured by using the informed consent document that outlines in very understandable terms the proposed treatment, stating the research is voluntary at all times.
- *Principle of beneficence:* Individuals must be protected from harm. Research should minimize risks and maximize benefits with a

clear explanation in the informed consent materials.

In addition to appropriate ethical conduct by researchers and physicians, patients must also follow through on *their* commitment to the study, insuring accurate data collection and ultimately protecting individuals who may use the therapy in the future.

In summary, prescription drugs would not be available without volunteer research participants and there are plenty of good reasons to participate in clinical research, beyond the obvious benefit to science. When deciding if a research trial is for you, it is important to understand that, although everything is done to insure the safety of research participants, the true safety and benefit of experimental treatments are not yet known. Knowing you may make a difference can be a very empowering way to participate in your own care.

MEDICINE FACTS & MYTHS

Myth: Levodopa stops working in 5 years. Fact: Levodopa does not stop working. In advanced stages, certain symptoms do not respond to dopaminergic medicines including levodopa.

Myth: Use of levodopa should be put off as long as possible. Fact: Levodopa is the best medicine for movement with lowest side effect. Levodopa is associated with dyskinesia especially at high doses so daily dose should be only what is needed.

Myth: The last medicine added is responsible for a new side effect. Fact: All dopamine medicines cause similar side effects but to varying degree. All medicines should be evaluated to determine which is more commonly associated with a side effect.

Alter Your Course

1. Scientific evidence proves PD is caused by a combination of genetics and environment. You, your lifestyle and the environment you live in can make a difference. Learn what is within your power to make a positive difference.

2. Parkinson's is a progressive condition. Although each person's condition is different, there are similarities in how symptoms progress. Use your knowledge of how symptoms typically progress and put a plan in place to combat these problems, i.e. target speech, motor coordination, balance, endurance, stress, depression and cognition.

3. Be aware of how your reaction to the diagnosis impacts your activities and attitude. Recognize that you have a choice in how you respond and this choice can include the decision to focus on the positive steps you can take rather than getting stuck in a negative reaction to what you have lost. You control the path you choose

4. Plan your journey with attention to knowledge, support, medical care, lifestyle, attitude and compassion.

5. Be an active member of your health care team and strive for the best results. Prepare for appointments, organize your healthcare data, set goals and assemble your team.

6. **Medications are an important part of your treatment, balancing neurotransmitter levels and setting the stage for enhanced movement. An optimal approach is individualized and balances the risks and benefits of medications.**

DEEP BRAIN STIMULATION

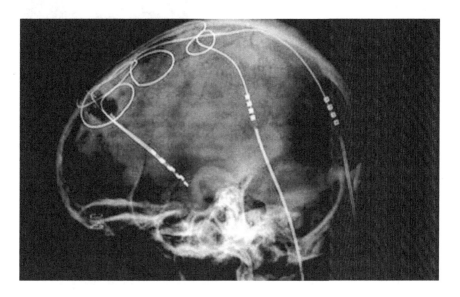

Renewal through electricity

Deep brain stimulation (DBS) is a surgical treatment for PD tremor, dystonia, motor fluctuations and dyskinesia. This neurosurgical procedure is not typically recommended during early stages of PD. Nonetheless, there are unique situations that prompt earlier consideration of DBS. Learning about DBS now before you need this therapy will help you make the right decision about surgery when needed and at the right time.

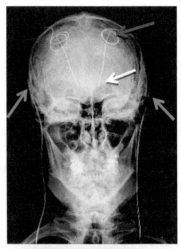

The surgical procedure involves implanting tiny wire(s) into the brain. The wires have four small electrodes that deliver customized continuous electrical impulses to regions deep in the brain. A neurostimulator (also called battery or generator) provides the power to send the impulses along the wire. The neurostimulator is implanted outside the brain usually under the collarbone.

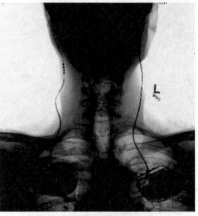

DBS lead wires are implanted into specific target regions or clusters of nerve cells called nuclei in the basal ganglia. You will remember that dopamine nerve cells are decreased in a specific region of the basal ganglia. Resultant changes in electrical firing of neurons located in this complex circuit of nerve cells are

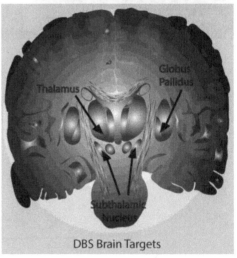

DBS Brain Targets

associated with PD motor symptoms. Electrical stimulation of two targets in this circuit, the subthalamic nucleus (STN) and globus pallidus interna GPi) influence patterns of nerve cell firing ultimately improving PD motor symptoms.

The best time for DBS therapy varies and is best understood through a discussion of risks and benefits.

In mild or early stage PD, levodopa or dopamine enhancing medications effectively improve motor symptoms throughout the day. Movements are often controlled with little to no variability (variability is called fluctuation) in response to each dose. In fact, many people do not notice that their next dose is due and must make special efforts to take medication on schedule. Of course people with Parkinson's can still have 'good' and 'bad' days or find that their symptoms change in situations associated with stress, fatigue or illness. DBS has not traditionally been recommended at this stage since medicine is effective and the risk of brain surgery outweighs the potential benefit. If symptoms are mild, the effects of DBS may not be very noticeable, yet the person will have to live with an implanted device that requires skilled medical professionals to provide device and stimulation oversight.

Sometimes tremor can be difficult to treat even when medication improves other movement symptoms. Additionally, patients with young onset PD may have difficulty with dystonia and/or dyskinesia during the early stages of PD. These symptoms can be associated with muscle pain and discomfort and may limit activities such as exercise, intimacy and sleep. Some people describe an underlying tension in the muscles that persists despite medication that contributes to emotional unrest and insomnia.

Deep brain stimulation is very effective for these potentially very disabling symptoms of tremor, dystonia and dyskinesia. Pain, muscle spasm and sleep quality can also improve. Deep brain stimulation is considered earlier for these specific symptoms if they are disabling despite adequate medication trials.

There is ongoing research that may shine more light on whether DBS should be considered in earlier stages of PD. If DBS were to slow some aspects of progression, then perhaps the benefit would outweigh the risk of having brain surgery. The decision to have DBS earlier comes down to risk. The most important question at this stage – *Are my symptoms bad enough or bothersome enough to justify the risks of brain surgery and have I tried the appropriate medication?*

Deep brain stimulation is most effective when medications still work yet the effect wears off before the next dose or when dyskinesia limits further medication increase. Stimulation improves the same symptoms that improve with medication. *An important point to remember is that symptoms that do not improve with dopaminergic medication (levodopa) do not typically improve with stimulation.* In other words, DBS is as *good as medication* but the effect of stimulation does not wear off like medications. The difference between stimulation and medication is that stimulation allows for smoother control of symptoms, less reliance on medication, less medication side effects, less dyskinesia, less tremor and less medication costs.

Deep brain stimulation is associated with risk. For example, cognitive changes and walking difficulty can occur after DBS surgery. Who will experience these changes is difficult to predict. Given the many factors that influence outcome a team approach with neurological, surgical and programming expertise is important for long-term success.

It is important that you do not feel pressured to have DBS. DBS surgery is not without serious risk of bleeding in the brain although rare, death can occur from brain surgery. Until we have proven data to support early DBS is beneficial for disease modification, the risk outweighs the benefit in early disease.

Note: This chapter is modified from the book *DBS A patient guide to deep brain stimulation.*

Alter Your Course

1. Scientific evidence proves PD is caused by a combination of genetics and environment. You, your lifestyle and the environment you live in can make a difference. Learn what is within your power to make a positive difference.

2. Parkinson's is a progressive condition. Although each person's condition is different, there are similarities in how symptoms progress. Use your knowledge of how symptoms typically progress and put a plan in place to combat these problems, i.e. target speech, motor coordination, balance, endurance, stress, depression and cognition.

3. Be aware of how your reaction to the diagnosis impacts your activities and attitude. Recognize that you have a choice in how you respond and this choice can include the decision to focus on the positive steps you can take rather than getting stuck in a negative reaction to what you have lost. You control the path you choose.

4. Plan your journey with attention to knowledge, support, medical care, lifestyle, attitude and compassion.

5. Be an active member of your health care team and strive for the best results. Prepare for appointments, organize your healthcare data, set goals and assemble your team.

6. Medications are an important part of your treatment, balancing neurotransmitter levels and setting the stage for enhanced movement. An optimal approach is individualized and balances the risks and benefits of medications.

7. **DBS is a treatment of mid-stage disease. Earlier DBS can be considered for medicine refractory tremor, dyskinesia or dystonia, especially if these symptoms are limiting exercise or sleep. An interdisciplinary team with specialized expertise can help you get the best results.**

NONMEDICAL THERAPIES

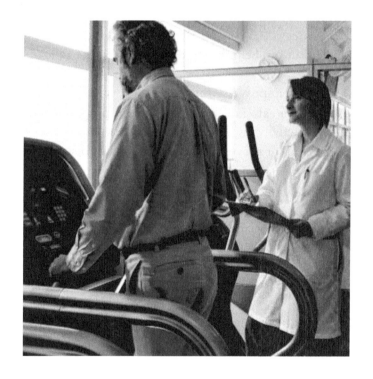

Exercise as Medicine

A proactive approach involves rehabilitation early before symptoms limit activities. This is especially important if you are considering changing your routine, giving up tasks, hobbies or exercise because of difficulties caused by your symptoms.

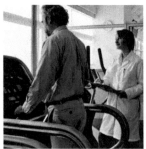

Posture, walking, coordination, balance, joint pain, speech and swallowing problems can improve with rehabilitation. Physical, occupational and speech therapy are an important part of your treatment. Traditionally rehabilitation is used to treat problems after they occur or significantly impact daily functions.

Rehabilitation can help during early stages in the following ways:

- Reduce or improve symptoms
- Establish a safe and targeted exercise program based on health, current activity level and symptoms
- Delay and/or prevent future symptoms of disease progression
- Establish optimal life strategies, habits, and goals
- Enhance work and home related chores

Rehabilitation specialists can also treat many non-motor symptoms or medication side effects as noted below:

- Sleep
- Fatigue
- Pain
- Bladder control
- Communication
- Dizziness
- Leg swelling
- Apathy

The following worksheet lists problems or goals that rehabilitation and other allied health providers can help you achieve. Items of particular importance early in disease are highlighted.

Rehabilitation Worksheet

Complete this worksheet to learn how rehabilitation may help you. Ask your neurologist for a referral to a specialist if you are experiencing any of the problems noted below.

** Additional copies of this form can be printed from the Holistic Brain Health Blog, www.drgiroux.com. **

Physical Therapy: Specializes in physical movement such as posture, joint pain, muscle flexibility and strength, balance and mobility, and provides exercise programs targeted to combat disease.

　　__**I need an exercise program specifically for my PD**
　　__**I am ready to increase my exercise level and activities**
　　__**I have pain that limits my activities or mobility**
　　__I get out of breath easily when walking or feel tired most of the day
　　__I have trouble getting out of a chair, car or bed
　　__I am having trouble with walking, falling or fear of falling
　　__I have problems with freezing while trying to walk
　　__**My posture is changing**
　　__I need a walking aid such as a cane or walker
　　__**I have exercise limitations**
　　__My care-partner needs information how to help me move
　　__**I have joint or muscle pain or spasms**
　　__I have problems with coordination
　　__I have trouble with bladder control
　　__I have mobility issues that keep me from going out
　　__I feel dizzy when I move
　　__I have lost power in my legs or tire easily
　　__I cannot stand for very long
　　__I fall or have a fear of falling

Occupational Therapy: Specializes in upper body function, dexterity, self-care, medication management, daily activities, driving, transportation, and resources for independence.

　　__**I have hobbies or home activities that are more difficult**
　　__**I have trouble at work with writing or typing**
　　__**I have problems completing tasks or organizing my day**
　　__**I am experiencing shoulder, neck or arm pain**

__I need more information on how to organize my medications
__I need help or have more difficulty with dressing or bathing
__**Tasks are taking longer**
__**I have fatigue, pain, weakness, coordination or thinking problems**
__**I need help with tasks, chores, work or hobbies**
__I have trouble with my vision
__I have problems with freezing while trying to walk
__I am fearful of falling or fall often
__I need help with home safety
__**I need help reviving my hobbies or other social interests**
__**I need a workplace evaluation**
__I have trouble getting out of bed, chair or car
__I need help with preparing a meal
__I have trouble sleeping or moving in bed
__I am concerned about driving or have transportation problems
__**I have motivation problems that affect my participation in daily activities**
__**My hobbies or work require coordination, dexterity or balance**

Speech Therapy: A comprehensive speech and voice evaluation is completed by a speech language pathologist. Therapy can help voice symptoms, swallowing difficulties, conversation and communication problems.

__I have problems swallowing food, liquid or pills
__I need to know which foods to avoid due to my swallowing problem
__I have lost more than ten pounds without trying recently
__I have excessive drooling and/or cough when I eat or drink
__I choke or worry about choking
__**I have problems with my speech**
__**I have problems being heard or difficulty communicating**
__**I have word finding problems**
__**Communication is an important part of my job**

Nutrition Consult: A registered dietician is trained to provide diet and nutritional counseling to improve nutrition, weight control, cholesterol, low and high blood pressure, leg swelling and diabetes.

__I am having trouble eating food due to a swallowing problem
__**I am having trouble maintaining or gaining weight**
__My meals are interfering with my medications
__I have food sensitivities, gluten sensitivity or celiac disease

__I have diabetes or kidney disease

__I experience bowel problem or constipation

__I am gaining weight

**__I have weight related problems: sleep apnea, joint pain, exercise
intolerance or fatigue with activity**

Psychology/Neuropsychology Evaluation: Specializes in the evaluation
of mood changes, adjustment, anxiety and support or thinking.

**__Treatment has improved my symptoms but I am having trouble
adjusting to my diagnosis**

__I am having trouble with anxiety of depression

__I am overly worried about my future

__I have confusion, memory problems, or problems making decisions

__I have more days feeling down that feeling good

__I have anxiety that interferes with my day to day activities

__I have thoughts or concerns that keep me awake at night

__My caregiver seems to be on edge, worried, or depressed

Social Work Evaluation: Provides emotional support, community
resources and adjustment with an emphasis on quality of life.

**__I need help finding what resources are available in my
community**

__I have questions regarding in home care or housing

__I am a carepartner in need of respite care

**__I am interested in attending a support group for carepartners
or patients**

__I have interests I would like to pursue but unsure where to start

__I need help with coping

__I am having trouble communicating with others

__I am feeling overwhelmed

Alter Your Course

1. Scientific evidence proves PD is caused by a combination of genetics and environment. You, your lifestyle and the environment you live in can make a difference. Learn what is within your power to make a positive difference.

2. Parkinson's is a progressive condition. Although each person's condition is different, there are similarities in how symptoms progress. Use your knowledge of how symptoms typically progress and put a plan in place to combat these problems, i.e. target speech, motor coordination, balance, endurance, depression and cognition.

3. Be aware of how your reaction to the diagnosis impacts your activities and attitude. Recognize that you have a choice in how you respond and this choice can include the decision to focus on the positive steps you can take rather than getting stuck in a negative reaction to what you have lost. You control the path you choose.

4. Plan your journey with attention to knowledge, support, medical care, lifestyle, attitude and compassion.

5. Be an active member of your health care team and strive for the best results. Prepare for appointments, organize your healthcare data, set goals and assemble your team.

6. Medications are an important part of your treatment, balancing neurotransmitter levels and setting the stage for enhanced movement. An optimal approach is individualized and balances the risks and benefits of medications.

7. DBS is a treatment of mid-stage disease. Earlier DBS can be considered for medicine refractory tremor, dyskinesia or dystonia, especially if these symptoms are limiting exercise or sleep. An interdisciplinary team with specialized expertise can help you get the best results.

8. Rehabilitation therapy is often overlooked in early PD. Ask for a referral to a rehabilitation specialist and focus on treatment, prevention and lifestyle change.

Alter Your Course

78

MOVEMENT &
NEUROPERFORMANCE
CENTER

COMPLEMENTARY THERAPIES

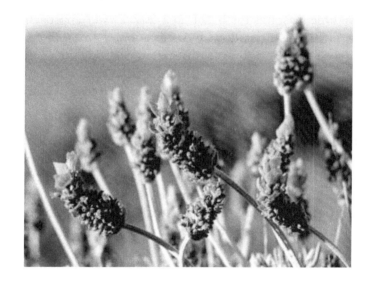

A holistic approach to health and healing

More people are searching for natural and alternative therapies to replace or complement traditional medical treatment. It is estimated that up 40-60% of Americans use alternative therapies for health and over 60% of people with PD have tried an alternative therapy. Observational studies found that 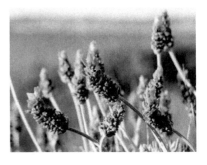 vitamins, massage therapy and acupuncture are the more commonly used complementary and alternative therapies (CAM) used in PD.

There are many reasons why people turn to CAM therapies after diagnosis. One reason is the belief in a *'more natural'* approach fearing the side effects associated with medication. Some are seeking a greater sense of control over disease and future progression by engaging in a holistic approach to target problems when medicines are not effective, while others wish to enhance a sense of balance and tap into their body's innate healing potential.

Integrative medicine represents a holistic approach embracing a philosophy of care that treats disease and personal wellbeing by combining traditional disease-oriented treatment with therapy that supports mind, body and soul; further supporting self-healing. By now you are already aware of the value of an integrative approach as the following findings support:

- **Activity:** Exercise improves PD symptoms and leads to positive neuroplastic brain changes.
- **Food:** Reduced risk of PD is associated with Mediterranean diet and increased risk with diets high in meat (saturated fats.)
- **Environment:** Pesticide exposure in the water, air or present in our food source are associated with increased risk of PD.
- **Emotions:** Stress not only worsens symptoms such as tremor but also directly impacts cellular health and physiology.

Complementary therapies are part of a holistic approach. Research studies analyzing the effect of these therapies is limited, seldom controlling for the placebo effect and rarely studying their long-term affect or impact. Nevertheless, the use of these therapies are gaining popularity and support from mainstream medicine.

The following complimentary therapies are summarized using categorization originally set forth by the National Center for Complementary and Alternative Medicine (NCCAM). Note: A complete discussion of complementary and holistic therapies for PD is beyond the scope of this chapter. You can learn more about holistic therapies and how to best integrate them into you medical care in the companion book, *Healing Parkinson's: A Holistic and Integrative Medicine Approach* (see reference section.)

Biological and Nutritional Therapy

Biological therapies include the medical benefits of food, nutritional supplements, herbs and plant based chemicals. Use of vitamins and supplements are the most common form of alternative therapy used by American's. Yet there is little evidence to date to suggest that these pills are effective in preventing or delaying neurologic disease in the absence of deficiency. Early results reporting benefit from glutathione injections, the supplement coenzyme Q10 and vitamin E in PD have now been repeated with disappointing results. Benefits at best are symptomatic and mild; and no supplement is proven to be more effective than traditional medicines nor proven to be neuroprotective. However, it is important to note that research studies evaluating the effect of nutritional supplements are very difficult to do, are usually performed over a short time period and studies analyzing long-term results are needed.

Vitamin D is commonly deficient in PD. As a neuro-hormone, vitamin D does more than enhance bone health. Lower levels are associated with poorer cognitive health and increased falls. Low vitamin D levels are measured at diagnosis and interestingly these levels do not decline further with disease progression. At present there is no data to suggest that increasing vitamin D levels with supplements changes the course of PD but is an important area of brain research.

Vitamin D should not be considered benign. Supplements, like medicines, can have serious side effects. High dose vitamin D supplementation without close follow-up can lead to serious effects. Excessive vitamin D levels can cause calcification in body tissues other than bone, a condition that can hasten atherosclerosis or vascular disease. A simple blood test can help you and your healthcare provider determine what dosage is best for you and follow the effects of vitamin D supplementation.

The following is a description of proposed mechanism of actions defining treatment categories listed in the following table.

- Antioxidants: Agents that reduce the cell damaging effect of oxidative stress, a byproduct of cell metabolism and proposed cause of nerve cell death in PD.

- Anti-inflammatory: Agents that reduce cellular inflammation, a proposed cause of nerve cell death in PD.

- Bioenergetics: Agents that enhance faulty cell energy production or serve as a brain or muscle energy source.

- Immune and neurochemical modulation: Agents that interact with our brain's immune health or circadian body rhythms.

- Micronutrients: Nutrients or trace elements required in small quantities to orchestrate a range of physiological function

- Neurochemicals: Agents that are precursors to neurotransmitters used by nerve cells.

- Natural Dopamine: Plants or derivatives that contain levodopa or dopamine.

- Herbals/Plants: Chemical derivatives or plant based agents with chemical properties used for their symptomatic properties.

The following table lists the more common vitamins and supplements used by people seen in consultation in our clinic and their potential mechanism of action.

Most Common Vitamins and Supplements

Proposed Mechanism	Supplement
Antioxidants	Vitamin E, C, Glutathione, N-Acetyl- Cysteine
Anti-Inflammatory	Fish oil, Omega 3 Fatty acids, Turmeric
Micronutrients	Calcium, Magnesium, Selenium, Vitamin B12, Folate, Thiamine or Vitamin B complex
Bioenergetics	Coconut oil, NADH, Coenzyme Q10, Creatine
Immune Modulators	Vitamin D, Melatonin
Neurochemical	Melatonin, SAMe, Tyrosine, 5-Hydroxy-tryptophan, Naltrexone
Natural Dopamine	Fava Beans, Mucuna Pruriens
Herbals/Plant	Marijuana, St. John's Wort, Chamomile, Lemon Balm, Ginger, Ginseng, Valerian Root

As stated earlier, there is no research evidence that confirms disease is improved with vitamins or supplements unless there is a noted deficiency (examples include vitamin B12 in vegetarians, or folate in pregnancy.) Yet numerous studies support the beneficial effect of <u>diets high in a particular vitamin</u> such as vitamin B12 in cognitive decline, vitamin B6 in Parkinson's disease, and folate in depression. There are likely many reasons why vitamins and nutrients ingested from food is more effective than pills including:

- Other coexisting vitamins or chemical agents found together in food work synergistically for health.

- People with a diet a high in a particular vitamin or supplement may pay greater attention to their overall health, eat a healthier diet and live a healthier lifestyle.

- Negative chemical and hormonal reactions occur as a result of rapid absorption into the bloodstream leading to abnormally high peaks in concentration rather than more controlled absorption when in their dietary form.

- Chemical structure of vitamins are sometimes similar to but not the same or in the same proportion as that found naturally in foods.

Where vitamins and supplements fail, a focus on a healthier diet succeeds in reducing risk of many diseases. Many diets are popular amongst PD individuals such as gluten- free, low carbohydrate and paleolithic diets. The Mediterranean diet is the only diet to date associated with reduced risk of PD and other brain diseases such as stroke, depression and Alzheimer's disease. We will focus on the role of diet and Parkinson's in the *Lifestyle* chapter.

Many people search for natural or herbal substances in place of standard pharmaceutical therapy. Fava beans contain a small amount of levodopa but levels vary significantly in beans. Favism is a form of anemia that can be a side effect in some people. Mucuna pruriens or cowhage seeds were first used to treat PD by Indian physicians practicing traditional Ayurvedic medicine over 400 years ago. The benefit of cowhage seeds is due to the fact that these seeds contain 3-4% levodopa. Research reporting benefit are limited (a placebo controlled trials studied only 8 patients) so we are left with little guidance in their use. Issues associated with product purity, consistency and potency are also a concern.

Body Therapy

Body therapies include exercise, massage, chiropractic and other forms of physical manipulation. *Exercise is no longer considered an alternative therapy as it should be a part of each person's treatment plan.* Some forms of exercise are unique in their focus on mind-body awareness or use of music and dance. More information on exercise is included in the lifestyle chapter. Examples of body therapies or exercise programs with potential beneficial results include:

Aerobic Exercise	Improved stamina, energy, cognition, weight management, diabetes and heart health, reduced movement symptoms and possible neuroprotective effects
Yoga	Balance, posture*, strength, mood, pain and emotional wellbeing
Tai chi	Balance, posture*, strength, mood, pain and emotional wellbeing
Dance	Balance, posture*, strength, mood, pain, social engagement and emotional wellbeing
Music Therapy	Bradykinesia, balance, posture*, strength, mood, and emotional wellbeing
Feldenkrais®, Alexander® Techniques	Balance, posture*, strength, mood, pain and emotional wellbeing

*Improved posture can directly improve speech volume.

The role of chiropractic manipulation and massage in PD is unclear. Anecdotal reports do suggest that these therapies can help pain, muscle spasm and anxiety. These therapies are usually delivered as part of a more holistic program combining the anti-stress effects of therapeutic touch and an environment that has a calming effect (i.e., music, aromatherapy and low ambient lighting) further enhancing perceived benefit.

Mind-Body Therapy

Mind-body medicine focuses on the premise that our mind and body does not breathe, move, feel, sense and perform in isolation but functions as a greater whole. Mind-body therapy uses techniques and experiences that integrate and engage emotional, mental, social and spiritual factors.

Mind-body therapies are used to reduce stress, reduce motor symptoms, improve general wellbeing and sense of balance. Stress reduction alone can help symptoms of PD. The following patient account describes how stress can impact disease.

"My dystonia (muscle spasm) and tremor are always worse at work. I find that I need to take extra medicine during the week. I need less medicine on the weekend since I am not bothered by my tremor on the weekend when I can relax and unwind."

The fact that stress makes tremor worse further supports the fact that your mind, experience and environment will influence your symptoms and therefore possibly effect treatments. Think about the impact of stress on your own symptoms. The key is to recognize when stress is present, how it affects you and techniques you can use to reduce the impact of stress.

The placebo effect is yet another example of how the power of the mind can change how you feel. The placebo effect (sugar pill) is a treatment effect not associated with the treatment itself but the power and belief that a treatment will work. The placebo effect in PD increases in proportion to the expectation that treatment will help.

Our attitudes, expectations and thoughts influence not only how we feel but also the outcome of treatments (traditional or complimentary).

Examples of mind-body therapies that can reduce stress, enhance emotional wellbeing, reduce symptoms and enhance the effects of treatments include:

- Meditation
- Mindfulness
- Hypnosis
- Breath Work
- Guided Imagery
- Music and Art therapy
- Nature based therapy

- Aromatherapy
- Movement therapy- Yoga, Tai chi, Feldenkrais®

Energy Medicine

Energy medicine is divided into veritable energy (measurable) and putative energy (not measurable) and works on the premise that energy systems exist in our body and their balance affects health. Blockage of these energies or energy in disequilibrium impacts disease. Energy waves from the environment can have a calming or energizing effect and also impact equilibrium, health and disease. Sound, visual, electromechanical, touch and emotional energy are examples of energy forms that are thought to promote healing. The strongest evidence of energy medicine and disease is the beneficial effect of full spectrum light therapy on seasonal depression. Examples of energy medicine include:

- Veritable (measurable)
  - Vibration Therapy
  - Magnet Therapy
  - Light Therapy- full spectrum light (sunlight) with UV filter effective for seasonal depression
  - Sound therapy
- Putative (yet to be measured)
  - Reiki
  - Qi Gong
  - Healing Touch
  - Acupuncture

Whole Systems Medicine

Acupuncture is gaining acceptance as a legitimate therapy in many pain conditions including headache and musculoskeletal pain. Its role in PD is still to be determined. Acupuncture is often performed as part of a more holistic traditional Chinese medicine approach (TCM). Whole systems approaches such as TCM and Ayurvedic medicine are centuries old and based on the premise that our body is a complex interdependent system in which health of a single organ (i.e. brain) requires that the body (at the cellular, chemical, or energy level) and organ systems must function in harmony with our emotions, spirit and the environment. Other healing practices such as faith healing and Native American healing remind us that our health is connected to a larger existence; connecting body, mind, spirit and the earth.

Practical Tips for Holistic Care

A practical approach is recommended for anyone interested in using CAM therapies given that there is limited research data to guide the use of these therapies in PD. The following recommendations can serve as a guide but are not a substitute for a conversation with your healthcare provider.

- Discuss the use of complementary therapy with your healthcare provider.

- Be sure to weigh the risk of a therapy when deciding on its use. Some therapies are lower risk such as massage therapy while others such as intravenous therapies are more invasive and carry greater potential side effects.

- Cost of these therapies can be high and often are not covered by insurance. Consider the effect of cost as you would any treatment related side effect. Be sure that you have the resources and that you are not limiting your ability to afford other necessities.

- Remember the placebo effect can result in over a 30% improvement in PD symptoms and is influenced by how much you expect something to work and how much value you attach to a specific treatment. Just because it worked for someone else does not mean it is the best treatment for you. Look for products and therapies that have been studied in a manner that controls for this effect.

- Focus on life-long lifestyle improvements such as nutrition, physical activity, emotional health and stress management over *'quick fixes'* found in a pill.

- Beware of flashy advertising and claims of a miracle cure. If the claims are too good to be true- that is probably true.

- Just because something is described as 'natural' or an herbal does not mean it is safe, effective, free of contamination or effective.

- Understand that supplements and vitamins can interact with your current prescription medicines. For example, St. Johns Wart, fish oil, garlic, vitamin E, and ginkgo biloba are examples of supplements that can interact with the blood thinner warfarin and increase risk of bleeding. *St. Johns Wort should not be taken with rasagiline (Azilect®.)*

- Remember that vitamins, supplements and herbal products are not FDA regulated like pharmaceutical drugs. Impurities, lack of potency and false labeling does occur. Look for products that are tested for purity, potency and bioavailability (how it is absorbed by the body) by an independent laboratory. This insures accurate and unbiased reporting. For instance, using products that carry 'USP' (United States Pharmacopeia) verification increases confidence of the potency and purity of the supplement or compound. This independent laboratory tests the purity, potency and bioavailability of products. In effect, this test insures that what is on the bottle label is indeed what is contained in the pill or supplement. Otherwise the actual purity and strength of the substance is not be reliable. The website <u>Consumerlab.com</u> is one resource to compare brand names.

Alter Your Course

1. Scientific evidence proves PD is caused by a combination of genetics and environment. You, your lifestyle and the environment you live in can make a difference. Learn what is within your power to make a positive difference.

2. Parkinson's is a progressive condition. Although each person's condition is different, there are similarities in how symptoms progress. Use your knowledge of how symptoms typically progress and put a plan in place to combat these problems, i.e. target speech, motor coordination, balance, endurance, depression and cognition.

3. Be aware of how your reaction to the diagnosis impacts your activities and attitude. Recognize that you have a choice in how you respond and this choice can include the decision to focus on the positive steps you can take rather than getting stuck in a negative reaction to what you have lost. You control the path you choose.

4. Plan your journey with attention to knowledge, support, medical care, lifestyle, attitude and compassion.

5. Be an active member of your health care team and strive for the best results. Prepare for appointments, organize your healthcare data, set goals and assemble your team.

6. Medications are an important part of your treatment, balancing neurotransmitters and setting the stage for enhanced movement. An optimal approach is individualized and balances the risks and benefits of medications.

7. DBS is a treatment of mid-stage disease. Earlier DBS can be considered for medicine refractory tremor, dyskinesia or dystonia, especially if these symptoms are limiting exercise or sleep. An interdisciplinary team with specialized expertise can help you get the best results.

8. Rehabilitation therapy is often overlooked in early PD. Ask for a referral to a rehabilitation specialist and focus on treatment, prevention and lifestyle change.

9. **A thoughtful blend of complementary therapies can enhance traditional treatment through personal healing, wellbeing and counter the negative impact of stress on disease.**

NEUROPROTECTION & NEUROPLASTICITY

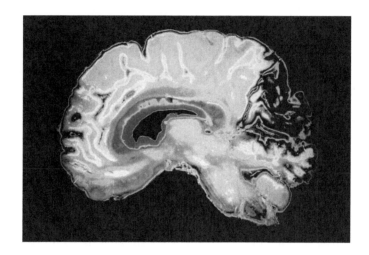

You can change your brain

Neuroplasticity is defined as the ability of brain cells and neural networks (nerve cell interconnections that form brain circuits) to change or modulate their connection and activity in response to activities and experiences. Nerve cells 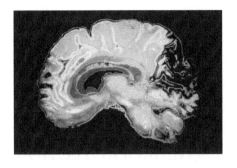 have interconnections that form circuits that are part of large networks. In essence, neuroplasticity allows the brain (and our senses, thoughts and body) to respond, adapt, understand, learn and modulate brain activity and performance in response to the needs and changes placed on us by our environment, activities and experience. These adaptations are possible due change in neural interconnections that expand networks to support change in brain activity.

It is important to remember that neuroplasticity is a constant process that allows us to learn, adapt and change. Neuroplasticity, then, can lead to both positive and adaptive or negative and maladaptive changes- depending on stimulus associated with how we live, think and behave.

Examples of maladaptive neuroplasticity include changes in brain connectivity and neurochemistry that lead to anxiety, depressed mood or post-traumatic stress disorder as a result of chronic exposure to a difficult environment, traumatic events or negative thoughts. Inactivity, lack of physical, cognitive or creative challenges can also alter brain activity and negatively impact physical and cognitive performance.

How we live life, our thoughts, attitudes, experiences and activities will impact our brain's function. This is a phenomenon that all people with PD can use to their advantage to shape their future.

There are many experiences and activities that drive positive neuroplastic change and it is not too surprising to learn that many of the same activities that improve quality of life also promote positive neuroplasticity. In other words, our brains have developed to respond in ways that further help us get the most out of activities that improve our quality living. We can consider positive neuroplasticity as a goal of therapy or treatment; whether it is the beneficial effect of medicine on the ability to move, a focused exercise plan or exposure to emotionally positive events.

There are many theories about what activities are most important and effective in promoting these positive changes. The following principles or qualities are important to drive neuroplasticity:

- Learning- New and innovative tasks, thoughts or activities that require us to learn new skills or ideas

- Complexity- Tasks that require attention, practice, and challenge

- Intensity- Actions that require increasing energy, work or practice

- Positivity- Activities that enhance positive feelings or attitude, sense of possibility and control

- Meaning- Activities that have powerful or personal meaning and significance

Additional factors that further influence the impact of these activities on neuroplasticity are:

- Repetition- Performing an action again and again

- Specificity- Choosing activities similar to the skill or performance desired

Physical

Since PD is associated with movement symptoms and changes in dexterity, agility and mobility, it is not surprising that exercise constitutes the area of greatest interest when it comes to neuroplasticity. We all know that exercise is good for our general health, strengthening our heart, muscles and body. Now we appreciate the added benefit of exercise when it comes to brain health and function. Exercise can enhance brain function and PD symptoms, motor performance and disease in the following ways:

- **Neuroplasticity**- Enhanced neural connections leading to improved physical performance and reduced impact of motor symptoms on motor performance. Reduction or delay in changes in symptoms over time associated with disease progression or aging (i.e., agility, coordination, power and balance.)
- **Neuroprotection**- Direct impact of physical activity on brain changes associated with disease. Although still an active area of study, therapeutic exercise may protect or minimize damage to vulnerable dopaminergic nerve cells at risk for degeneration.

We all know that exercise is good for us and now understand there are brain positive benefits of exercise. *So what exercise is best and how much should be done?* This question is addressed in the lifestyle chapter, but the following observations gleaned from brain research serve as a foundation and encouragement to help you begin or enhance your exercise program.

Something is better than nothing!

Functional brain imaging shows an increase in brain activity over the motor cortex (cell area on the surface of the brain dedicated to the control of movement) after just minutes of practice, sometimes as little as 10 to 15 minutes.

This finding reminds us of the importance and positive impact of practice on brain activity, even for a short period of time. Many people with Parkinson's say that they do not have enough time or are too tired to exercise as noted in the following patient's discussion:

"I do not have enough time to go to the gym and exercise. Even half an hour is hard to find in my busy day. Plus I am too tired to even think of exercising."

If this scenario sounds all too familiar, remember the powerful impact of exercise on how you feel and the fact that even a few minutes can make a difference. Over time, symptoms, mood, stamina and energy will improve reinforcing your motivation to increase time dedicated to exercise. Set aside a few minutes in the day to exercise or practice a task that is bothering you such as handwriting, speech (speaking loudly) or balance- even if it is only for a brief duration of time. Daily practice will give you the best response and this helps build helpful habits to offset the impact of some PD symptoms.

Practice makes perfect

An Olympic athlete will train over and over again to improve performance to an extreme level. Performing a task over and over again will improve brain function through strengthened or new nerve cell connections and this will ultimately improve performance. You do not have to be an Olympic athlete to benefit from practice. Focused repetition of a task or skill will improve performance at any level of ability or disability. This is the idea behind the 'forced use' physical therapy technique first pioneered in stroke rehabilitation. Forced use was noted to improve arm weakness and the ability to perform daily tasks otherwise compromised due to weakness. In this form of physical therapy, the patient's good arm is restrained 'forcing' the weaker arm to do everyday tasks such as dressing, eating, phone and computer work. Research confirms that brain activity, hand strength and function are improved with this therapy when compared with standard physical therapy.

Talk to your doctor about medication if you notice PD affecting one side of your body, especially if you are not doing certain activities because of symptoms. For example, you may be right handed and now find that you are using your left hand to do more activities such as dressing, eating or writing. Loss of coordination and strength are a consequence of disuse and inactivity. Medication can help improve symptoms so that you can improve movement. Consult with an occupational therapist to see if changes in treatment, targeted exercise or strategies can be put in place to help you use your affected side better. Targeted exercises can restore and maintain a more normal movement of an arm or leg that is impacted by PD.

Repetition is not the only important training principle. As the term *practice* implies, it is important to focus on 'normalizing' movement just as an Olympic athlete would focus on perfecting performance. Many therapy programs incorporate exercises designed to counteract motor changes brought on by altered basal ganglia physiology associated with PD. Exercises can be tailored to exaggerate amplitude, power, posture, balance and flow of sequential movements (what is referred to as therapeutic exercise.)

Aerobic and endurance activities may be important!

Aerobic exercise that is physically challenging may be especially helpful. Researchers studied the effect of 'forced exercise' on rodents subjected to a neurotoxin designed to destroy dopamine nerve cells. These animals display parkinsonian-like movement changes and represent an animal model used to investigate potential treatments. Rodents 'forced' to exercise on a running wheel showed less degeneration in dopamine nerve cells (and less decline in motor control) after injection with the neurotoxin when compared to more sedentary animals.

This finding, called neuroprotection, suggests that exercise can 'protect' dopamine nerve cells otherwise vulnerable to further degeneration associated with disease. Similarly, intensive aerobic exercise can improve motor symptoms such as tremor and speed of movement in people with PD. Ongoing studies are investigating the possible causes of these changes including altered brain neural activity, efficiency of dopamine use by nerve cells or nerve terminal sprouting.

More than Just Movement

You have already learned that PD is more than just a movement disorder with cognitive, behavioral, sensory and autonomic nervous system changes. Some non-motor symptoms such as cognitive abilities, sleep and mood impact quality of life and in some situations are more bothersome than motor symptoms.

The best PD therapy includes a holistic approach treating non-motor problems in concert with motor symptoms. Similarly, research and observations on neuroplasticity suggest a holistic approach is especially effective when it comes to brain activity. This includes activities that challenge non-motor performance. Neuroplasticity is further enhanced by activities that carry a positive meaning such as:

- Activities that are complex and challenging
- Activities that integrate movement, senses and emotions
- Activities with personal meaning, purpose or spiritual growth
- Activities focused on positive thoughts, emotions and experiences

Quality not just Quantity!

The quality of exercise, activity or experience is just as important as intensity. Once again, rodent studies offer insight to this important concept. Creative and challenging exercises are designed where rodents are exposed to a colorful and diverse 'jungle gym.' This more creative and enriched exercise environment increases nerve cell connections in the cerebellum (motor coordination and control region of the brain) when compared to rats exposed only to a running wheel. This observation was noted even though rodents exercised much longer on the running wheel compared with the jungle gym- *quality not quantity.*

These principles can also explain why balance is improved when music, dance and laughter is included as part of an exercise routine when compared to balance exercises alone.

Meaning and Positivity

Quality of exercise includes more than the challenge of adding activities that combine cognitive-sensory-motor integration. The emotional *'meaning'* and personal significance we apply to an experience is also important. For example, the neuroprotective effects of exercise is reduced when parkinsonian rodents are exposed to a stressed environment one in which sleep wake cycle is altered, diet is changed and animals are isolated from their litter mates. Of course these experiments cannot be performed with people but do suggest that our environment- whether positive or negative- is important. The impact of meaning and the quality of your experience is also significant as is highlighted through observations that the impact of exercise differs whether performed in a group, is an activity you enjoy or experienced in nature versus indoors.

Holistic Activity Holistic Effects

Finally, as alluded to above, movement is a complex integration of motor, sensory, emotional and cognitive processes. Our mood affects our movement, movement affects our mood and our thoughts affect our performance. Engaging and integrating these multiple systems may lead to enhanced neural activity and further integration of these functions at the cellular level.

A holistic approach to neuroplasticity and brain health with and without disease will have a broader impact. Be sure to:

- Add diversity to your routine
- Focus on more than movement
- Reduce the impact of stress
- Explore activities that add meaning, joy, purpose and value

Alter Your Course

1. Scientific evidence proves PD is caused by a combination of genetics and environment. You, your lifestyle and the environment you live in can make a difference. Learn what is within your power to make a positive difference.

2. Parkinson's is a progressive condition. Although each person's condition is different, there are similarities in how symptoms progress. Use your knowledge of how symptoms typically progress and put a plan in place to combat these problems, i.e. target speech, motor coordination, balance, endurance, depression and cognition.

3. Be aware of how your reaction to the diagnosis impacts your activities and attitude. Recognize that you have a choice in how you respond and this choice can include the decision to focus on the positive steps you can take rather than getting stuck in a negative reaction to what you have lost. You control the path you choose.

4. Plan your journey with attention to knowledge, support, medical care, lifestyle, attitude and compassion.

5. Be an active member of your health care team and strive for the best results. Prepare for appointments, organize your healthcare data, set goals and assemble your team.

6. Medications are an important part of your treatment, balancing neurotransmitter levels and setting the stage for enhanced movement. An optimal approach is individualized and balances the risks and benefits of medications.

7. DBS is a treatment of mid-stage disease. Earlier DBS can be considered for medicine refractory tremor, dyskinesia or dystonia, especially if these symptoms are limiting exercise or sleep. An interdisciplinary team with specialized expertise can help you get the best results.

8. Rehabilitation therapy is often overlooked in early PD. Ask for a referral to a rehabilitation specialist and focus on treatment, prevention and lifestyle change.

9. A thoughtful blend of complementary therapies can enhance traditional treatment through personal healing, wellbeing and counter the negative impact of stress on disease.

10. **Capitalize on the positive effects of neuroplasticity with experiences and activities that offer challenge, meaning and positivity.**

EMOTIONAL WELLBEING

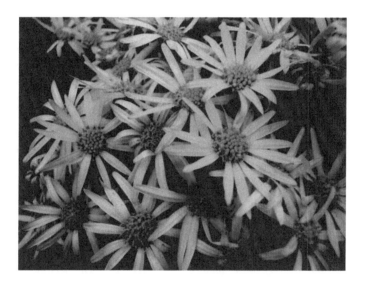

Social , creative and nature experiences may be protective against depression and anxiety

Photo by Sierra Farris

Depression and anxiety can be one of your very first symptoms or occur at any time after diagnosis. Recognition and treatment of mood changes is very important since your thoughts, attitude and mood, will influence how you feel, perceive your world and ultimately

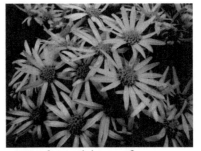

experience life with PD. Depression can replace visions of possibility with visions of hopelessness, sadness, insecurity, and impossibilities ultimately impacting the decisions you put in place after you hear the phrase, *"you have Parkinson's disease."*

Research confirms that depression impacts quality of life as much or more than motor symptoms reinforcing the importance of your emotional wellbeing and personal outlook on how you feel today and into the future. Treat your emotional well-being with the same level of importance as you would your movement symptoms.

Look beyond medicines and exercise as your primary treatment. These therapies will be even more successful if your attitude and mood are positive, expanding your thoughts and activities to the power of possibility rather than the power of negativity that can accompany the worry of disease.

Depression

Depression is a medical condition. Up to 50% of people with PD experience symptoms of depression sometime during the course of PD. Depression has many causes. It can be a primary problem independent of PD (this usually is associated with a history that extends to early adulthood). Depression can also be a symptom of PD, caused by other medical conditions or medications. The observation that depression often occurs before the first motor symptoms suggest that depression is a PD symptom caused by neurologic and biochemical changes in neurotransmitters that influence mood such as serotonin, dopamine, and norepinephrine.

Depression is a psychological response. Depression is also caused by our thoughts, experiences, circumstances, worries, social isolation, loneliness or frustrations when symptoms cause problems with everyday tasks. Symptoms of depression include sadness, memory problems, fatigue, sleepiness or altered sleep habits. Other symptoms of depression include irritability, poor concentration, loss of enjoyment in activities and hobbies, social withdrawal, change in appetite, decreased libido, feeling of hopelessness or guilt, excessive worrying, feeling of worthlessness or failure and suicidal thoughts. Apathy or loss of motivation and anxiety can coexist with depression.

Depression affects you and your family's well-being in many ways. Remember, the better your mood, the more likely you will tend to your 'wellness' routine with exercise, healthy eating, adapt to your difficulties, problem solve and socialize with people important to you. The statement below describes a person's experience with mild tremor and illustrates how depression affected her perception of disease, treatment and future outlook:

"My tremor is really bad. Everything is so difficult. I am too tired to do anything but go to work and when I come home all I can do is lay on the couch. I feel like my disease is progressing very fast and there is nothing I can do about it."

Anxiety

Anxiety is experienced as nervousness, excessive worrying, feeling jittery, having an unsettled mind or inability to stop thoughts that interfere with daily activities or sleep. Anxiety can limit concentration and attention, social interactions and worsen symptoms of PD. Common physiologic changes associated with anxiety include palpitations, racing pulse, sweatiness, jitteriness, shortness of breath, atypical chest pain, nausea, loss of appetite, muscle tightness (especially in the neck, shoulder and trunk), and headache.

Anxiety is a medical condition. Anxiety can occur from changes in brain regions that influence mood and is a common symptom of PD.

Anxiety is a psychological response. Anxiety can be part of your 'worries' about diagnosis, your future, finances or other life concerns. It can be constant or change with your fluctuating motor symptoms.

For example, in mid-stage, feelings of anxiousness can occur when Parkinson's medications wear off prior to the next dose. Certain movement symptoms can increase or worsen with anxiety, especially tremor, dystonia and gait freezing (a problem in later stages of PD.) Some people with PD describe phobias or situations that are associated with anxiety such as fear of crowds.

When anxiety is tied to your movement problems, one problem can worsen the other, like a *snowball effect*. This may sound familiar to you if you have tremor and experience an increase with stress or anxiety. Anxiety can even influence how your medicines will work for you either limiting the benefit or increasing side effects.

You can feel well with Parkinson's! **

Depression and Anxiety are Treatable

There are many personal and lifestyle changes you can take to understand and improve emotional changes associated with PD. Given the many factors that impact mood, anxiety or stress, a multifaceted approach is best. The following list includes examples of activities or therapies that may be helpful.

- *Medication:* Anti-depressants and anti-anxiety medicines can be helpful, especially if biochemical changes are involved.
- *Medical Conditions:* Treating associated problems such as heart disease, sleep apnea, pain conditions and thyroid disease can improve mood.
- *Behavioral counseling:* These therapies are administered under the guidance of a psychologist, psychiatrist, counselor, social worker or other mental health provider. Counseling helps identify feelings, mood or stress triggers and offer strategies or steps to combat problems, adjust to change and manage fears. Cognitive behavioral therapy (CBT) is proven helpful for PD. This technique explores the many conditioned negative thoughts we may not be aware of that lead to increased anxiety, depression or hopelessness in a challenging situation. Through CBT you can learn to recognize these thoughts and triggers and replace them with more positive or productive thoughts and strategies to

improve mood, reduce stress and enhance how you ultimately respond to problems.

- *Lifestyle therapies:* Aerobic exercise, healthy eating, adequate sleep, creative expressions, experiences with nature, and social contact with family, friends and loved ones are very important steps not to be overlooked.
- *Positivity:* Keeping your environment positive is important. Focus on what you can rather than what you can't do. Even simple changes such as exposure to people or situations that make you laugh can make a difference.
- *Care for your carepartner:* Be sure to include your carepartner as this person is also at risk for depression
- *Healing and relaxation:* Therapies such as acupuncture, therapeutic yoga, massage and Reiki can improve mood and anxiety.
- *Mindfulness and stress reduction:* Mindfulness therapy works on the premise that:

  - A physiologic balance exists in our bodies between the state of relaxation and stress.
  - Our thoughts, judgments and reactions in the moment influence how we feel.
  - We can tailor our response to our environment, emotions or bodily sensations through a practice of bringing awareness to the moment and influence our judgmental reactions.
  - Examples include: mindfulness therapy, guided imagery and meditation

More information on mind-body therapy and mindfulness can be found at www.drgiroux.com.

The information above is educational only and should not take the place of professional care and guidance.

Alter Your Course

1. Scientific evidence proves PD is caused by a combination of genetics and environment. You, your lifestyle and the environment you live in can make a difference. Learn what is within your power to make a positive difference.

2. Parkinson's is a progressive condition. Although each person's condition is different, there are similarities in how symptoms progress. Use your knowledge of how symptoms typically progress and put a plan in place to combat these problems, i.e. target speech, motor coordination, balance, endurance, depression and cognition.

3. Be aware of how your reaction to the diagnosis impacts your activities and attitude. Recognize that you have a choice in how you respond and this choice can include the decision to focus on the positive steps you can take rather than getting stuck in a negative reaction to what you have lost. You control the path you choose.

4. Plan your journey with attention to knowledge, support, medical care, lifestyle, attitude and compassion.

5. Be an active member of your health care team and strive for the best results. Prepare for appointments, organize your healthcare data, set goals and assemble your team.

6. Medications are an important part of your treatment, balancing neurotransmitter levels and setting the stage for enhanced movement. An optimal approach is individualized and balances the risks and benefits of medications.

7. DBS is a treatment of mid-stage disease. Earlier DBS can be considered for medicine refractory tremor dyskinesia or dystonia, especially if these symptoms are limiting exercise or sleep. An interdisciplinary team with specialized expertise can help you get the best results.

8. Rehabilitation therapy is often overlooked in early PD. Ask for a referral to a rehabilitation specialist and focus on treatment, prevention and lifestyle change.

9. A thoughtful blend of complementary therapies can enhance traditional treatment through personal healing, wellbeing and counter the negative impact of stress on disease.

10. Capitalize on the positive effects of neuroplasticity with experiences and activities that offer challenge, meaning and positivity.

11. **Pay as much attention to your emotional health as you do your movement symptoms. Your emotional wellbeing can impact quality of life as much or sometimes more than motor symptoms.**

MOVEMENT &
NEUROPERFORMANCE
CENTER

LIFESTYLE

EXERCISE AND DIET

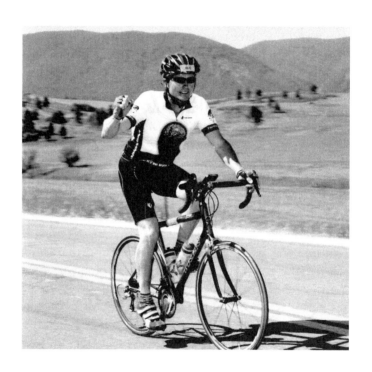

-Photo courtesy of John Carlin, Thriving with PD

This chapter expands upon on the importance of exercise and nutrition introduced in prior chapters.

Exercise

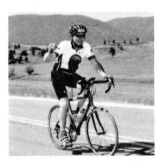

As you have learned exercise can improve your physical and emotional health, motor performance, stamina, cardiopulmonary function, and can combat physiologic brain changes associated with PD. Exercise will positively impact your future health further instilling a sense of control, resiliency, ability to adapt and hope.

Exercise will also enhance brain function to complement your restored movement. *Exercise has the potential to reduce or delay the impact of problems such as flexed posture, weakness, fatigue and imbalance that can worsen with age or disease progression.*

Keep in mind that your prior activity level will guide your exercise program. Your muscles, connective tissue, heart and lungs will need a progressive exercise routine to challenge you. In other words, your exercise routine will expand as your fitness improves. A physical therapist can help you begin or expand your exercise program to reduce injury and improve performance. Professional guidance is especially helpful if your symptoms limit movement or cause pain. Setting and modifying goals that are within reach every four to six months will allow you advance your routine, stay motivated and experience increasing benefit over time.

Other symptoms can dictate the exercise that you do, such as apathy, depression, imbalance, arthritis, high or low blood pressure, diabetes, heart or lung disease and fatigue. Talk to your doctor or health care provider about a referral to a physical therapist or an exercise physiologist to get started on a safe program. These professionals will work with you to monitor and advance your routine so that you are safe, do not get injured, stay on track and are successful with your program.

Exercise – The Evidence and Practice

What is exercise? Exercise is any activity that is purposeful, moves the body and/or activates the brain. As you have learned neuroplasticity takes place when learning is a component of the exercise and this finding has moved this important PD treatment to the forefront.

Is exercise harmful? Debunking an old myth!

Just a decade ago, many thought exercise was harmful for people with PD speculating that perhaps exercise 'used' the dopamine reserves otherwise available for movement. Dr. Giselle Petzinger debunked this myth upon publishing her research on exercise and neuroplasticity. To summarize her findings:

- Exercise does not cause a change in dopamine cell number
- Exercise does not change total amount of dopamine but increases dopamine release from nerve cells
- Dopamine is used more efficiently by the brain with a decreased rate of turnover
- Exercise decreases glutamatergic activity in the basal ganglia (a good thing)
- Dopamine and glutamate changes are important for normal basal ganglia function.

Collectively, this information provides us with compelling evidence that intensive exercise can alter basal ganglia neurotransmission and promote recovery in people with PD.

What is the evidence?

What is the best exercise for PD? This is a common question that arises in clinic. There is no single exercise that is 'best' for PD as these research findings suggests:

- Moderate intensity exercise improves absorption of levodopa.
- Exercise reduces dyskinesia.

- Qi Gong improves non-motor symptoms including constipation, pain and sleep.
- Strength training improves power, endurance, mobility and reduces fall risk.
- Aerobic exercise improves gait and fitness.
- High intensity strength training improves mobility, leg power and slowness.
- Treadmill training improves walking, reduces fall risk and improves quality of life.
- Tai Chi improves gait and balance and reduces fall risk.
- Progressive strength training improves motor symptoms.
- Tango and Foxtrot improves mobility.
- Respiratory muscle training improves sense of shortness of breath.
- Mental power and imagery can increase muscle strength without moving a muscle.
- Moderate exercise can change the brain and improve motor symptoms.
- Vigorous exercise appear to lower the risk of developing PD.

Considering the complexity and adaptability of brain physiology and function, it is not surprising that a balanced and multi-faceted approach will gain the broadest benefit. For example, an exercise program combining twice weekly aerobic, strength training, stretching, balance, water exercises and gymnasium activities improved PD motor symptoms, mood, wellbeing, fitness, strength, coordination, motor skills and flexibility after only 14 weeks.

Exercise does more than improve the physical and motor aspect of PD. Exercise can improve executive function commonly associated with PD and even brain size. Aerobic exercise can improve executive skills such as task planning and execution, problem solving, attention, abstract thinking and reasoning. Aerobic exercise also prevents brain cell loss or the tendency toward decreased brain size with aging, a process that can be associated with cognitive deficits.

Exercise will also greatly impact how you feel, move and perform. As Dr. Giroux commonly reinforces with patients, *"you are going to feel only as well as your general health allows."* Regular light to moderate exercise will improve bone density, blood glucose, cholesterol, and blood pressure, heart, and lung function. The increase in muscle mitochondria density, leg strength and power that occurs with regular and challenging exercise will improve energy levels and stamina- both a common problem with advancing PD.

Exercise for Specific PD Symptoms (based on published research)

Gait	Tango, Tai chi, Treadmill, Strength training, Aerobic exercise
Balance	Tango, Tai chi, Treadmill, Strength training,
Tremor	Aerobic, Mindfulness based movement
Rigidity	Tango, Aerobic, Cross training
Slowness	Tango, Aerobic, Cross training, Music therapy
Cognition	Aerobic
Mood	Aerobic, Strength training, Intensive cross training, Yoga
Sedation, Pain, Constipation	Qi Gong

Exercise Principles & Safety

Exercise guidelines are available on the internet but do not replace oversight by your healthcare provider. The authors subscribe to physical activity and exercise recommendations provided by the American College of Sports Medicine (ACSM.org). A visit with your primary physician and physical therapist is important before starting or increasing your exercise intensity. An exercise specialist who is certified in the field of exercise testing, exercise risk factor mitigation and exercise prescriptions for clinical conditions can also help. Caution is highly advised when accepting only the advice of a personal trainer as their credentials (if any) do not meet the standards to work with a person with a neurological condition unless supervised by a certified exercise specialist, physical therapist or healthcare provider. These conditions require physician supervision prior to an exercise program: *uncontrolled heart arrhythmia, symptomatic orthostatic hypotension or uncontrolled blood pressure, severe aortic stenosis, uncontrolled heart failure, acute pulmonary embolism, acute myocarditis, dissecting aneurysm or acute or ongoing chest pain.*

These factors are considered when designing an exercise program:
- Safety Factors such as balance and impulsivity
- Medications
- Risk Status
- Exercise Capacity – requires exercise testing
- Cognition and Mood Factors – requires physician input
- Orthopedic (bone and joint) Limitations and Osteoporosis
- General Health and Medical Problems - such as blood pressure, heart disease and diabetes
- Exercise History
- Personal Health & Fitness goals

Special attention should be given to PD medications and side effects, gait, freezing, balance, fall risk, mental status, sensory and autonomic function, deep brain stimulation, motor fluctuations, dyskinesia, dystonia, neck and spine status and bladder function.

An effective and safe exercise program should start low and progress in intensity for optimal response. Professional guidance can ensure you are on the right track and that the intensity is increased appropriately as your performance improves. With exercise, more is not always better. For instance, exercising every day may seem like a good idea but the rate of injury greatly increases with more than 4 intensive days a week. Remember however that this does depend on intensity and type of activity. For instance, walking can be done every day. Keep in mind that a varied and balanced exercise routine will get broader results and potentially minimize injury.

Exercise intensity is generally measured by your perception of exertion and this is closely linked to heart rate. For instance an individual's perception that they are exercising vigorously usually is associated with the upper limits of achievable heart rate that can be sustained during exercise. People with PD can have a blunted perception of exercise intensity in moderate to advanced stages and can have a blunted response in heart rate to exercise. If perceived exertion is blunted, you may need to work with your exercise specialist to define alternative methods to monitor exercise exertion (not based solely on percentage of estimated maximum heart rate.)

Program Examples from Research Paradigms

Research studying aerobic (treadmill or cycling), strength training or balance training shows benefit when performed two to four times a week over a 4 to 16 week period. Measured benefits from dance, Tai Chi and Qigong were noted in studies ranging from 2 to 12 months with sessions range from 30 to 90 minutes. Overall the benefits of exercise in PD can occur within one month, a time course similar to people without PD. The physical gains of exercise diminish within two months reinforcing the need for a life-long commitment.

Exercise Guidelines

Take the Physical Activity Readiness Questionnaire from ACSM before beginning an exercise program or starting a new physical activity. If you answer yes to any of the following questions, you should seek medical advice prior to engaging in a physical activity or exercise program.

1. Has your doctor ever said that you have a heart condition and that you should only do physical activity recommended by a doctor?
2. Do you feel pain in your chest when you do physical activity?
3. In the past month, have you had chest pain when you were not doing physical activity?
4. Do you lose your balance because of dizziness or do you ever lose consciousness?
5. Do you have a bone or joint problem that could be made worse by a change in your physical activity?
6. Is your doctor currently prescribing drugs (example, water pills) for your blood pressure or heart condition?
7. Do you know of any other reason why you should not do physical activity?

ASCM exercise guidelines established include 150 minutes per week of moderate-intensity physical activity. With PD, an additional focus should include balance, agility, posture, respiratory muscles, gait, visuospatial, dual task and learning.

ACSM Recommendations for Physical Activity (see acsm.org)

Cardiorespiratory Exercise

- Work up to 150 minutes of moderate-intensity exercise per week.
- Strive to exercise 30-60 minutes of moderate-intensity exercise over 5 days/week or 20-60 minutes of vigorous-intensity 3 days/week.
- Multiple shorter sessions (of at least 10 minutes) are acceptable to accumulate exercise time.
- Gradually increase exercise time, frequency and intensity for adherence and to reduce risk of injury
- Any activity is better than no activity.

Resistance or Strengthening Exercise

- Exercise major muscle groups 2-3 days a week.
- Very light or light intensity is best for older adults or adults with chronic conditions when starting exercise.
- Complete at least 2 sets of each exercise for strength and power.
- Complete at least 8-15 repetitions improve strength and power, and 15-20 repetitions for muscular endurance.
- Wait at least 48 hours between strength training sessions.

Flexibility Exercise

- Complete 2 or 3 days each week to improve range of motion.
- Hold each stretch should for 10-30 seconds to the point of tightness.
- Repeat each stretch at least twice, accumulating 60 seconds per stretch.
- Slow and controlled stretching is recommended. No pain should occur.
- Complete flexibility exercise only after the body has completed a warm up of light aerobic activity or a hot bath to warm the muscles.

Neuromotor Exercise

- Neuromotor exercise (called "functional fitness training") is recommended 2 or 3 days a week.
- Motor skills (balance, agility, coordination and gait), proprioceptive exercise training and multifaceted activities (Tai chi, Yoga, Qigong).
- Incorporate 20-30 minutes per day.

Other

- Sitting for long periods of time should be avoided.

Staying Motivated

Motivation is an important part of starting and sticking with your regular exercise routine. Consider keeping an exercise calendar in a highly visible place such as the kitchen. This daily reminder of your goals and progress will inspire motivation and *fan the fires* of determination. Begin by setting easy and obtainable short-term goals to keep you moving forward toward your ultimate goal. Set out your exercise clothing in advance for the day. If you feel lackluster energy to exercise, simply put on the exercise gear and the urge to get moving may soon take over. Setbacks happen when there is company, family events, vacation, days when you are not feeling well or are injured. Setbacks can be viewed as the speed bumps in life that are just part of living. They may slow you down periodically but not halt you in your tracks. Don't internalize unnecessary stress when you experience a break from your exercise routine. All that is truly important is that you make the effort and commitment to resume your routine when possible.

Exercise Nutrition

Remember, to fuel the body for exercise you need to drink plenty of water, eat healthy and snack often if participating in endurance exercises. High energy but healthy food such as dried fruit, yogurt, nuts and seeds can keep you going and provide the healthy anti-oxidants so important for brain health. Be sure to discuss the use of supplements such as creatine, amino acids, sports drinks, etc. with your physician before use as they are not without side effects.

Nutrition

We are all aware that a healthy diet will reduce risk of heart disease, diabetes, cancer, high cholesterol and high blood pressure. What is less known is that diet can impact mood, cognition, fatigue, brain health and brain disease.

Our culture loves fad diets but fads come and go only to be replaced by the next. Just look on the internet or your local bookstore and you will find hundreds of diets proving instant health, weight loss or cures. Some limit entire food groups while others let you eat whatever you want. These easy 'fixes" do not promote long-term healthy lifestyles. On the other hand a balanced diet is a proven foundation for overall health and is here to stay.

A wholesome, balanced diet is not the typical American diet. The American diet has changed dramatically over the years with a focus on convenience and fast foods. The American diet is:

- High in fast food, convenience food and processed foods. Processing removes food and ingredients from their natural nutrient rich state. For example fruit roll ups made with 'real fruit' will never replace the nutritional and health benefits of fresh fruit.
- High in processed foods made with unhealthy trans-fats or hydrogenated oils, chemical preservatives, artificial color, sweeteners and high fructose corn syrup.
- Excessive in protein (and saturated fats) from non-plant sources.
- High in salt.
- High in chemical additives and artificial sweeteners.
- High in processed carbohydrates.
- Low in fruits and vegetables.
- Low in protein from beans, nuts and seeds.
- Low in high quality, unprocessed whole grains.
- Low in healthy oil from fish, seeds and nuts.

The link between food and health is undeniable. Of particular interest is the Mediterranean diet and its impact on health. The Mediterranean diet is associated with:

- Increased lifespan
- Lower incidence of obesity
- Improved glucose control and type 2 diabetes control
- Reduced risk of heart disease
- Reduced risk of cancer risk and increased cancer survival

The link between the Mediterranean diet and brain disease includes:

- Reduced risk of stroke
- Reduced risk of depression
- Reduced risk of Alzheimer's and...

- Reduced risk of **Parkinson's disease!**

The Mediterranean diet is low in processed convenience food and high in wholesome unprocessed foods. Features of this diet are:

- High in fruits and vegetables
- Meals low in red meat (less than 3-4 times a month)
- High in vegetable protein from seeds, nuts and beans
- High in fish at least twice weekly
- High in whole grains over processed and simple sugars
- High in fiber from whole grains, fruits, vegetables
- Olive oil in place of butter, margarine and other fats
- Garlic and other spices to enhance flavor without salt or sugar
- Red wine

Chemical features of this diet important for brain health include the high proportion of foods with antioxidants and anti-inflammatory properties. Anti-oxidants are chemical molecules that reduce the toxic effect of chemically reactive oxygen compounds produced by the body from cell metabolism. These highly reactive molecules can damage nerve cells, a process called oxidative stress. Oxidative stress is a proposed cause of cell death in Parkinson's and other brain disease. Inflammation is also a potential cause of brain disease including Parkinson's disease. Foods high in saturated, trans and hydrogenated fats and carbohydrates high in glycemic load increase cell inflammation. Foods with cellular and health promoting properties include:

- Anti-oxidants- Pigmented fruits, vegetables, seeds, nuts, beans, wine, spices. Choose foods rich in color and variety.

- Anti-inflammatory- Oils (omega 3) from fish, limited meat, carbohydrates from whole grains rather than processed or simple sugars

Constipation

Constipation can be a problem in early disease and can even precede motor problems as an early symptom of PD. A diet high in fiber (20-30g) from beans, fruits, vegetables and whole grains can help combat constipation. Be sure to drink plenty of water for colon health.

Protein

Protein is important for energy, muscle mass and cell growth. Protein can slow the absorption of levodopa in the intestine. For this reason, many people with PD reduce the amount of protein they eat or when they eat it. However, the impact of protein on levodopa absorption and symptom control is typically a problem later in disease when on-off fluctuations require strict timing of medicine and not as critical in early disease. However an awareness of how much protein you eat and when can help you later in disease if you are experiencing motor fluctuations.

Organic Foods

The cause of Parkinson's is not yet known but environmental factors are associated with an increased risk. An exposure to pesticides is the strongest link between the environment and an increased risk of developing PD. Eating organic foods can reduce ingestion of pesticides but organic produce is expensive. Be sure to wash all produce in warm water with mild soup if organic foods are not an option. Foods with thick skins of peels have lower pesticide levels. The Dirty Dozen and Healthy Fifteen are lists of foods (available on the internet) with higher and lower pesticide exposure; respectively, to help you choose which foods to eat organic.

Alter Your Course

1. Scientific evidence proves PD is caused by a combination of genetics and environment. You, your lifestyle and the environment you live in can make a difference. Learn what is within your power to make a positive difference.

2. Parkinson's is a progressive condition. Although each person's condition is different, there are similarities in how symptoms progress. Use your knowledge of how symptoms typically progress and put a plan in place to combat these problems, i.e. target speech, motor coordination, balance, endurance, depression and cognition.

3. Be aware of how your reaction to the diagnosis impacts your activities and attitude. Recognize that you have a choice in how you respond and this choice can include the decision to focus on the positive steps you can take rather than getting stuck in a negative reaction to what you have lost. You control the path you choose.

4. Plan your journey with attention to knowledge, support, medical care, lifestyle, attitude and compassion.

5. Be an active member of your health care team and strive for the best results. Prepare for appointments, organize your healthcare data, set goals and assemble your team.

6. Medications are an important part of your treatment, balance neurotransmitter levels and setting the stage for enhanced movement. An optimal approach is individualized and balances the risks and benefits of medications.

7. DBS is a treatment of mid-stage disease. Earlier DBS can be considered for medicine refractory tremor dyskinesia or dystonia, especially if these symptoms are limiting exercise or sleep. An interdisciplinary team with specialized expertise can help you get the best results.

8. Rehabilitation therapy is often overlooked in early PD. Ask for a referral to a rehabilitation specialist and focus on treatment, prevention and lifestyle change.

9. A thoughtful blend of complementary therapies can enhance traditional treatment through personal healing, wellbeing and counter the negative impact of stress on disease.

10. Capitalize on the positive effects of neuroplasticity with experiences and activities that offer challenge, meaning and positivity.

11. Pay as much attention to your emotional health as you do your movement symptoms. Your emotional wellbeing can impact quality of life as much or sometimes more than motor symptoms.

12. **Whether through neuroplasticity, physiologic brain changes, general health, mood or symptom control, your diet and exercise will impact your future with PD.**

FAMILY, RELATIONSHIPS & WORK

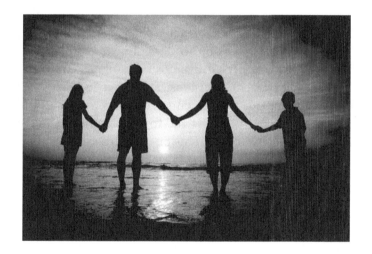

Alter your course!

Family and Relationships

How will your diagnosis change your relationships and your family?

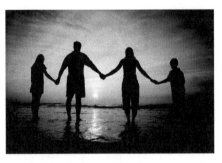

Relationships are bound to change after diagnosis. You may be surprised to learn that some couples and families describe changes for the better. Successful couples understand and prepare for the challenges of PD together and use the opportunity to prioritize time together, reconnect and strengthen their commitment or their personal relationships with friends and family.

Your family or partner will react to your Parkinson's disease in their own way and how they react will affect you. Some take on an early role as caregiver seeking to do as much as possible. They may deal with the uncertainty of diagnosis by taking control of medical appointments, treatment decisions, and lifestyle changes. They may be vigilant about your movements, carefully watching and noticing any change from day to day. If the focus is too great this may cause an added level of anxiety and tension The other end of the spectrum is the partner or family member that has difficulty coming to terms with the diagnosis. They may deal with uncertainty and fear by distancing themselves, not getting involved with medical appointments and/or treatment decisions. Still others take a middle of the road approach balancing their own involvement in a way that allows you, the person with PD, to stay in control with the benefit of their support.

There is no right or wrong approach. Like life itself, these reactions will change and mature over time. Of course how you and your family or partner react to life with PD is something that you will experience together. Talk about your diagnosis, emerging concerns and how you would like to handle your disease- as a couple or family.

Do you wish to have your partner involved in all aspects of your treatment? If so, how will this work out best for the two of you? Can you strike a balance so that this experience is positive, supportive and is shared by both?

Coming together around adversity can strengthen relationships and we have seen this to be true after diagnosis. Life is full of choices and this is an opportunity to prioritize and make choices based on what you value in life. Prioritizing your time with those most important to you can serve as a helpful anchor for the whole family when dealing with times of change and uncertainty.

Communication is an important part of any relationship and this is especially true when dealing with a chronic condition. Unique communication challenges for a person with PD include:

- Depression or apathy
- Masked facial expression or blunting spontaneous expression (referred to as mask-like face)
- Softer more monotone speech
- Decreased body language
- Social withdrawal

Friends and family may assume that you are not interested or invested in the moment. Educating them about these changes can help them understand that these problems can exist and are not reflective of your interest.

If you have young children at home you have probably struggled with the question, *should we tell the children?* Think about how this information would change your situation at home. Your children may already be aware of a change in your movement, sense a change in your mood or level of stress. Not knowing why can be a source of fear and anxiety. Having an open and honest discussion, at a level they can understand can help reduce those fears, and reinforce the strength of family especially if you and your partner present a united approach to this challenge. Remember to discuss your situation and concerns with your healthcare provider, family counselor, social worker or other behavioral health specialist for more support. Professional help can offer guidance especially since children will react in different ways and their understanding will depend on age and development.

Intimacy

There is a fine balance between bringing PD into your relationships and not letting it define your relationships. Remember to take the time to re-connect with your spouse or partner in a way that PD is not the entire focus. A counselor who is trained to help with coping strategies, the grieving process and relationship issues can help guide the discussion about what is working, what is missing and what is needed in the relationship. Think about the following discussion points. It might be helpful to sit down with your loved one and discuss these issues together in an open, honest and respectful manner.

- How has/will PD change our relationship?
- What can I do to make the relationship stronger? Are there opportunities to refocus, set new priorities and bring us closer together?
- What is working well and what needs more attention?
- Could we find some quality time each week where we sit, talk, listen and truly hear what the other has to say?
- What am I doing that is causing un-necessary stress on the relationship?
- Should we meet with a counselor for guidance?
- Are there different ways to connect emotionally, explore and experience intimacy?

If you are concerned about sexual intimacy, talk about it. This might even be an opportunity for you and your partner to connect on a greater emotional level. Make time for yourself and remember that intimacy is an important part of a relationship. Intimacy means different things for different couples. Taking the time to touch and reconnect on an emotional level keeps your relationship focused on the positives.

You may find that a discussion of sexual difficulties is given little to no priority at medical visits even though it may be on the top of your list of problems. If you find you are not getting enough attention, ask your doctor who is best suited to address and help you with this problem. Sexual health requires a multidisciplinary approach for the best results. Medical problems such as diabetes, hypertension, heart disease and some medicines can also affect sexual performance. Specialists that may help include gynecologists, urologists, sex therapists, counselors or your family doctor.

Sharing Your Diagnosis

With whom and when you should share your diagnosis is highly personalized and depends on many different factors. Before openly talking about the diagnosis, many people consider:

- The added stress on their children or parents
- Not being able to explain the many unknowns about PD
- Being treated differently by family, friends and peers
- Receiving too much attention due to the PD
- Losing a job, relationship or friendship
- Being misunderstood or left out
- Feeling vulnerable or being perceived as 'weak'

Ask your healthcare provider if there is a nurse, social worker or someone you can talk to about this topic. Learn how others with PD handled this situation and the results. If you are hesitant, you may find that some of your fears or worries are alleviated if you find a safe way to start talking about PD with your family and friends. The more you know about PD, the easier it will be to talk with others to alleviate their concerns for you. You are the same person, you just happen to have PD.

Workplace Issues

The average age for diagnosis is under 60 years old so many people have several years before retirement. Young onset individuals may just be hitting the peak in their career or are still raising children. No matter when the diagnosis hits, the financial implications and related work concerns are real.

Should I tell my boss and coworkers that I have PD?

There are pros and cons to informing your employer about your diagnosis. In an ideal situation you will spend less energy hiding your symptoms or worrying about being *found* out. You may find a sense of support, camaraderie and genuine kindness from your coworkers. Your positive take charge attitude may be seen as a great source of inspiration and admiration from your peers. Your boss and coworkers may work with you to find new ways to achieve your goals, perform difficult tasks and get the job done.

But, things can also turn out very differently. Your boss and coworkers could be inflexible and not very accommodating to your situation or show little to no commitment to make work a positive experience or even possible.

Consider the following before you make a decision about revealing your diagnosis at work:

- Is there a history of trust, culture of flexibility and innovation, camaraderie and teamwork?
- What is the economic and financial situation of your company?
- Are your skills and experience so unique that you are not replaceable?
- Do you have protections against being pushed out?
- Do you have disability insurance?

These are tough questions. Many organizations offer confidential counseling through an employee assistance program. Seek counseling outside the workplace if you are uncomfortable talking about your diagnosis with your employer. Know your rights and, if needed, consult with an attorney that specializes in disability, discrimination or workplace issues.

Is Disability Inevitable?

Make a list of the requirements of your job both today and into the future. The following list is not complete but illustrates one approach:

- Is the job physically demanding requiring a good deal of mobility, dexterity and stamina or is balance needed to climb ladders, etc.?
- Do you have primarily a desk job that requires you to multitask and be cognitively sharp throughout the day?
- Do you use the computer?
- Is driving required for work?
- Do you rely on specific talents such as drawing?
- Do you manage people or events?
- Do you enjoy your job, does it add a sense of self-worth or value to life, and does this override the stressors that come with work? Is the opposite true?
- Is public speaking or verbal communication an important part of your job?

Put a plan in place to help you stay on top of your job requirements. Talk to your healthcare provider about medications especially if your movement symptoms are not controlled, you are experiencing a wearing off of medication effectiveness or if you are experiencing side effects that can affect your performance such as sedation, thinking changes and impulsivity control.

Your rehabilitation team can help you manage, adapt and plan for the demands of work. An occupational therapist can help you with time and organizational management, setting up an efficient and ergonomic workstation, recommend adaptive aids and computerized gadgets to help you get the job done. A physical therapist can help if your job requires physical strength, stamina or balance. A speech therapist can help you with communication. A neuropsychology evaluation can help if you feel there is a change in attention and concentration, multitasking, planning or completing a task.

Work stress and its impact on you and your symptoms cannot be overstated. Until you have put a plan in place, the worry and stress of work related concerns can be overwhelming making it more difficult to focus. There are many stress management techniques that may fit your lifestyle and some have a dual purpose, such as yoga for relaxation, strength and balance or meditation for stress management, emotional wellbeing and clarity of thought.

Retirement

It is never too early to plan for retirement. Review all insurance policies such as life insurance, long-term care insurance and disability insurance. Are they adequate to protect you and your family? Can or should they be increased? These policies can be obtained after you have been diagnosed but may be much more expensive. A financial planner or accountant can help you analyze the benefit versus cost ratio of increasing or adding insurance. There are also organizations such as the American Association of Retired People (www. AARP.org) that can help you research your options.

If you are just facing retirement with a new diagnosis of PD, this is an opportunity to make this time work for you. Commit to a focus on positive lifestyle changes and social engagement. Often people retire from a lifelong job and experience a loss of self or identity. Don't replace work with TV. Instead add purpose, meaning and value to your life through volunteering, community involvement, spiritual activities and support of others. (Remember support groups are not just for you to get support but also for you to give support.)

Life Planning

Long term care planning, unlike other action items, includes planning for the worst case scenario and preparing for end of life. Although this may seem far off, being proactive and discussing the possibilities that you may face in the future is a positive step in avoiding a crisis later. This may include a change in your living arrangement. Does your home allow living on one floor in the event balance is a problem? Do you live alone? Do you have the support and resources to live at home if you need additional help?

Some people decide to make changes early further simplifying life and making positive decisions on a positive note before it is needed rather than a negative reaction to a crisis or being told they '*have to for their own safety*' by others. Others may decide to live closer to metropolitan areas to reduce distance driving and have access to more readily available services and activities. Moving may not be desirable or practical, but talking through these issues before there is a problem gives you and your family time to think about the best solution. When and if you will need more advanced care is unknown. Parkinson's is a slowly progressive condition so there is time to prepare and in most cases you will have a decade or more to prepare for the unknown. Making decisions under more urgent conditions is much more stressful.

Getting your health related documents in order is another aspect in long term care planning. Talk with your partner or family member about your wishes at end of life so these wishes will be known. The Family Caregiver Alliance offers additional information and guidance on these topics at www.caregiver.org. There are simple tasks that once completed, are there when you need them. The following documents are typically included in long term health care planning:

- *Durable Power of Attorney-* Legal document allowing you to give a person the authority to make financial and legal decisions for you in the event that you are incapacitated and not able to do so.
- *Health Care Proxy-* Legal document designating a person that will have the right to make healthcare decisions for you if you are incapacitated by illness or accident and not able to do so for yourself.
- *Advanced Care Directive-* A document prepared in advance, giving specific instructions about your healthcare wishes in the event that you are unable to do so and at end of life.

Make an appointment with your doctor or healthcare provider if you are recently diagnosed and uncertain about work issues, symptom impact or life planning.

Alter Your Course

1. Scientific evidence proves PD is caused by a combination of genetics and environment. You, your lifestyle and the environment you live in can make a difference. Learn what is within your power to make a positive difference.

2. Parkinson's is a progressive condition. Although each person's condition is different, there are similarities in how symptoms progress. Use your knowledge of how symptoms typically progress and put a plan in place to combat these problems, i.e. target speech, motor coordination, balance, endurance, depression and cognition.

3. Be aware of how your reaction to the diagnosis impacts your activities and attitude. Recognize that you have a choice in how you respond and this choice can include the decision to focus on the positive steps you can take rather than getting stuck in a negative reaction to what you have lost. You control the path you choose.

4. Plan your journey with attention to knowledge, support, medical care, lifestyle, attitude and compassion.

5. Be an active member of your health care team and strive for best results. Prepare for appointments, organize your healthcare data, set goals and assemble your team.

6. Medications are an important part of your treatment, balance neurotransmitter levels and setting the stage for enhanced movement. An optimal approach is individualized and balances the risks and benefits of medications.

7. DBS is a treatment of mid-stage disease. Earlier DBS can be considered for medicine refractory tremor dyskinesia or dystonia, especially if these symptoms are limiting exercise or sleep. An interdisciplinary approach with specialized expertise can help you get the best results.

8. Rehabilitation therapy is often overlooked in early PD. Ask for a referral to a rehabilitation specialist and focus on treatment, prevention and lifestyle change.

9. A thoughtful blend of complementary therapies can enhance traditional treatment through personal healing, wellbeing and counter the negative impact of stress on disease.

10. Capitalize on the positive effects of neuroplasticity with experiences and activities that offer challenge, meaning and positivity.

11. Pay as much attention to your emotional health as you do your movement symptoms. Your emotional wellbeing can impact quality of life as much or sometimes more than motor symptoms.

12. Whether through neuroplasticity, physiologic brain changes, general health, mood or symptom control, your diet and exercise will impact your future with PD.

13. **Be aware of how PD changes your family, work and other relationships. Seek the advice of family and career counselors when needed.**

MOVEMENT &
NEUROPERFORMANCE
CENTER

FINAL ADVICE
FROM THE TRENCHES

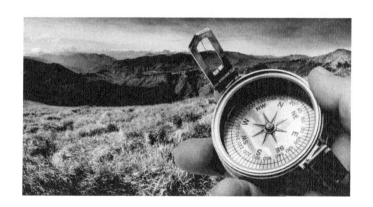

We have shared much of what we have learned from our patients with you in this book.

In this section we invited people *'in your shoes'* to share their advice.

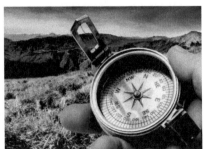

`We asked 10 people/partners living with PD to answer one of two questions.

1. What do you wish you had when you were diagnosed with PD (i.e. advice, information, support, what to do, what did or did not go well at the time of diagnosis)?

2. Using your own experience what advice would you give others just recently diagnosis?

We pass this advice on to you and your carepartner as a message of hope, inspiration, perseverance and courage.

"Never give up - this is the beginning of your journey. Here are a few suggestions for living well with Parkinson's: Try something - if it doesn't work - try something else. Keep flexible in mind and body. Being positive is a choice. Create a great support network. Stay active. Join a support group. Find what works for you, every day."

-Karl PD 20 yrs and Angela Care-partner 17 yrs.

"You can identify with the disease with a focus on your symptoms even before they ever occur. Alternatively, you can use diagnosis as a spring board for positive lifestyle and personal change. Changing my focus of attention in this way has helped me deal with the bad days and uncertainty."

-Janice PD 4 yrs.

"Do not let PD become you or swallow you up. This can happen if you overdo your focus on the disease. Take on a new, totally different challenge. One that packs a 'double whammy' by adding quality to your time and positivity to your life. For me that was cross country skiing, which had the added benefit of keeping me active and making me work on coordination and balance. Set your sights on a long-term goal that keeps you going throughout the years. For me that is completing a big cross country ski 20 times. Also remember that your symptoms will fluctuate day to day and this is natural so don't stress about these changes. Focus instead on long-term changes."

-Peter PD 11 yrs.

"I wish I believed in myself more at diagnosis. What I mean is that I did not feel that I had the strength and courage to look PD in the face and 'stare it down'. After a few years, I learned that I had what it takes to be strong. I found that strength by going to support groups and learning from others."

-Alison PD 7 yrs.

I wish I pushed myself early to get involved in a young onset group. I did join an online group and met my friend who has been there for me. Also, never give up hope. Always know that if something is not working, whether it be medication or DBS, there is always hope. Do not settle. If someone else is feeling hopeless, you may have to stand in and fill in the gap for them. Remind them to hold onto hope.

-Jessica YOPD 10 yrs

We all wish to go through our lives healthy and happy, but then something happens to shatter our lives in some way. First most of the time they are things that we can't prevent from happening. So you need to be strong and face this in the eye and fight it. Don't take the limitations that are handed to you from well meaning (doctors, family and friends) on how this is going to affect you personally as your condition progresses. Everyone is different, same thing in one person can effect someone else differently. I have found that you will able to do more than you or others thought, so push the Limits. I have a cup half full attitude. I enjoy photography and hiking. I will never stop living and 'Pushing the Limits' in life.

-Nathan PD 10 yrs.

Find one thing to be grateful about each day, whether big or small. This will help you keep things in perspective and not let PD become your life. -Richard PD 6 yrs.

My Advice, make friends with other people with PD. It will make all the difference in the world to have buddies with whom you can share this complicated; and at times demanding; emotionally and physically difficult journey. Find a movement disorder specialist who listens to you and is empathetic. Learn about your disease and make sure all your medical decisions are well informed. -Betsy PD 11 yrs.

The focus should be on the positive. How can you, with the help of your healthcare team, stay healthy so you can work on healthy perceptions of the disease in mind, body and spirit? What are ways that a combination of medicines, physical therapy, positive reading, family and other supportive people can help you take immediate and positive actions that will help you? -Mary PD 20 yrs.

Get involved. I hesitated at first but eventually joined a support group. I am not one to talk about my feelings much, but I found that I opened up to others at the group and felt more at ease.

-Jim PD 8 yrs

Alter Your Course

1. Scientific evidence proves PD is caused by a combination of genetics and environment. You, your lifestyle and the environment you live in can make a difference. Learn what is within your power to make a positive difference.

2. Parkinson's is a progressive condition. Although each person's condition is different, there are similarities in how symptoms progress. Use your knowledge of how symptoms typically progress and put a plan in place to combat these problems, i.e. target speech, motor coordination, balance, endurance, depression and cognition.

3. Be aware of how your reaction to the diagnosis impacts your activities and attitude. Recognize that you have a choice in how you respond and this choice can include the decision to focus on the positive steps you can take rather than getting stuck in a negative reaction to what you have lost. You control the path you choose.

4. Plan your journey with attention to knowledge, support, medical care, lifestyle, attitude and compassion.

5. Be an active member of your health care team and strive for the best results. Prepare for appointments, organize your healthcare data, set goals and assemble your team.

6. Medications are an important part of your treatment, balancing neurotransmitter levels and setting the stage for enhanced movement. An optimal approach is individualized and balances the risks and benefits of medications.

7. DBS is a treatment of mid-stage disease. Earlier DBS can be considered for medicine refractory tremor dyskinesia or dystonia, especially if these symptoms are limiting exercise or sleep. An interdisciplinary team with specialized training can help you get the best results.

8. Rehabilitation therapy is often overlooked in early PD. Ask for a referral to a rehabilitation specialist and focus on treatment, prevention and lifestyle change.

9. A thoughtful blend of complementary therapies can enhance traditional treatment through personal healing, wellbeing and counter the negative impact of stress on disease.

10. Capitalize on the positive effects of neuroplasticity with experiences and activities that offer challenge, meaning and positivity.

11. Pay as much attention to your emotional health as you do your movement symptoms. Your emotional wellbeing can impact quality of life as much or sometimes more than motor symptoms.

12. Whether through neuroplasticity, physiologic brain changes, general health, mood or symptom control, your diet and exercise will impact your future with PD.

13. Be aware of how PD changes your family, work and other relationships. Seek the advice of family and career counselors when needed.

14. **Remember you are not alone. Reach out to others and for help and support. Offer help and support, in kind, when you are able.**

SELECTED REFERENCES

Alcalay RN. Movement Disorders, 2012. 27: 771–774. The association between Mediterranean diet adherence and Parkinson's disease.

Beal MF. Annals of Neurology, 2003. 53: S39-s48. Bioenergetic approaches for neuroprotection in Parkinson's disease.

Caap, AM and D O. Aging Clin Exp Res, 2002 ,.4::371-7. Factors of importance to the caregiver burden experienced by family caregivers of Parkinson's disease patients.

Carter, J et al. Caregiver Role Strain in Parkinson's Disease: Diagnosis and Clinical Management. Factor SA, Weiner WJ. (eds). New York: Demos Medical Publishing; 2002.

Cheng EM, Swartztrauber K et al. Movement disorders, 2007. 22:525-522. Association of specialist involvement and quality of care for Parkinson's.

Choe MA. Korean Journal of Physiology & Pharmacology, 2012. 16: 305-312. Effects of Treadmill Exercise on the Recovery of Dopaminergic Neuron Loss and Muscle Atrophy in the 6-OHDA Lesioned Parkinson's Disease Rat Model.

Davis B. Clinical Nursing Research, 2005.14:253-272. Mediators of the relationship between hope and well-being in older adults.

Dufault S. Nursing Clinics of North America, 1985. 20:379-391. Hope: Its spheres and dimensions.

Egnew TR. Annals of Family Medicine, 2005. 3:255-262. The Meaning Of Healing: Transcending Suffering

Elbaz A et al. Journal of Clinical Epidemiology, 2002. 55: 25-31. Risk tables for parkinsonism and Parkinson's disease.

Grosset KA, Grosset DG. Movement Disorders, 2005. 20:616-619. Patient-perceived involvement and satisfaction in Parkinson's disease: effect on therapy decisions and quality of life.

Hirsch MA and Farley BG, 2009. 45:215-29. Exercise and neuroplasticity in persons living with Parkinson's disease.

Farry P et al. Postgrad Med Journal, 2002. 78:924 612-614. Use of complementary therapies and non-prescribed medication in patients with Parkinson's disease

Giroux ML and Farris SF. Topics in Geriatric Rehabilitation, 2008. 24: 83-89. Treating Parkinson's Disease: The Impact of Different Care Models on Quality of Life

Grosset KA, Grosset DG. Movement Disorders, 2005. 20:616-619. Patient-perceived involvement and satisfaction in Parkinson's disease: effect on therapy decisions and quality of life.

Grosset D et al. J Neurol Neurosurg Psychiatry, 2007. 78:465-469 .A multicentre longitudinal observational study of changes in self-reported health status in people with Parkinson's disease left untreated at diagnosis.

Helané Wahbeh ND, et al. Neurology, 2008. 70: 2321–2328. Mind-body interventions: Applications in Neurology

Herth K. Journal of advanced nursing, 1990.15:1250-1259. Fostering hope in terminally-ill people.

Hoehn M and Yahr MD. Neurology, 1967. 14:427. Parkinsonism: onset, progression, and mortality.

Kann M et al. Annals Neurology, 2002. 51: 621-625. Role of parkin mutations in 111 community-based patients with early-onset parkinsonism.

Kahn EJ. Neurol Neurosurg Psychiatry, 2012. 83:164-170. Deep Brain Stimulation in Early Stage Parkinson's Disease

Kübler-Ross, Elizabeth MD (1996-2004) was a Swiss American psychiatrist whose pioneering theory, 5 stages of grief was introduced in her 1969 book *On Death and Dying*, inspired by her work with terminally ill patients.

Lee MA, Walker RW, Hildreth AJ, Prentice WM. Movement Disorders, 2006. 21:1929-1934. Individualized assessment of quality of life in idiopathic Parkinson's disease.

McInerney-Leo, A et al. Movement Disorders, 2005. 20: 1-10 Genetic testing in Parkinson's disease.

Petzinger J et al. Lancet Neurology, 2013. 716-2622. Exercise-enhanced neuroplasticity targeting motor and cognitive circuitry in Parkinson's disease.

Rutten S et al. Parkinson's Disease, 2012. Online article. http://dx.doi.org/10.1155/2012/767105. Bright Light Therapy in Parkinson's Disease: An Overview of the Background and Evidence

Schrag A. et al. Parkinsonism & Related Disorders, 2002. 35-41. Caregiver-burden in Parkinson's disease is closely associated with psychiatric symptoms, falls, and disability.

Seifert, K and Wiener J. American Journal of Neurodegenerative Disease, 2013. 2: 29–34. The impact of DaTscan on the diagnosis and management of movement disorders: A retrospective study.

Shulman L et al. Movement Disorders, 2001. 16:507-510. Comorbidity of the nonmotor symptoms of Parkinson's disease.

Stewart, M., et al. The Journal of Family Practice, 2000. 49: 796-804. The impact of patient-centered care on outcomes.

Suchowersky O. Neurology, 2006. 66:976-982. Practice Parameter: Neuroprotective strategies and alternative therapies for Parkinson disease (an evidence-based review). Report of the Quality Standards Subcommittee of the American Academy of Neurology

Swarztrauber, K et al. Neurology, 2006. 6: 26. The quality of care delivered to Parkinson's disease patients in the U.S. Pacific Northwest Veterans Health System BMC

Swarztrauber, KE. Graf, et al. Movement Disorders, 2007. 22: 704-707. Nonphysicians' and physicians' knowledge and care preferences for Parkinson's disease.

Tillerson JL et al. Neuroscience, 2003. 119: 899-911. Exercise induces behavioral recovery and attenuates neurochemical deficits in rodent models of Parkinson's disease.

Vav der Marck. Parkinsonism and Related Disorders, 2009. 15 S3: 219-22. Multidisciplinary care for patients with Parkinson's disease.

Warner T, Schapira A. Annals of Neurology, 2003. 63: 818-826. Genetic and environmental factors in the cause of Parkinson's.

Veit C, Ware J. Journal of Consulting and Clinical Psychology, 1983. 51:730-742. The structure of psychological distress and well-being in general populations.

Weintraub D, Moberg PJ, Duda JE, Katz IR, Stern MB. Journal of the American Geriatrics Society, 2004. 52:784-788. Effect of psychiatric and other nonmotor symptoms on disability in Parkinson's disease.

Zhao Y et al. Movement Disorders, 2010. 25: 710-716. Progression of Parkinson's disease as evaluated by Hoehn and Yahr stage transition times.

MOVEMENT &
NEUROPERFORMANCE
CENTER

RESOURCES

Patient Information Blogs by Authors

www.DrGiroux.com

DrGiroux.com contains helpful tips to support better living with dystonia, tremor and Parkinson's disease with medication, lifestyle and wellness.

www.dbsprogrammer.com

DBSProgrammer.com contains important information about DBS.

Foundations
General Patient Information

American Parkinson's Disease Association, www.apdaparkinson.org

Northwest Parkinson's Foundation, www.nwpf.org

Davis Phinney Foundation, www.davisphineyfoundation.org

Michael J Fox Foundation, www.michaeljfox.org

National Parkinson's Foundation, www.parkinson.org

Parkinsons Disease Foundation, www.pdf.org

Advocacy

Parkinson's Action Network, www.parkinsonsaction.org

Caregiving

Family Caregiver Alliance, www.caregiver.org

ABOUT THE AUTHORS

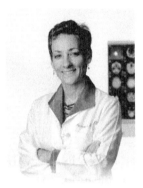

Monique Giroux, MD embraces a holistic approach to Parkinson's disease including medical, surgical, rehabilitative and integrative therapies with a focus on treating the person not just the disease. Dr. Giroux is the only U.S. Neurologist to complete fellowship training in Movement Disorders and Integrative Medicine. Her informative blog, unique with its focus on self-care and holistic health, educates people internationally. She is medical director of Swedish Medical Center Movement Disorders and DBS program in Englewood, CO, medical faculty for National Parkinson's Foundation's National Allied Team Training and medical director of the Northwest Parkinson's Foundation. She has experience and leadership in interdisciplinary care, extensive training in DBS management, Botox therapies, and mind-body medicine.

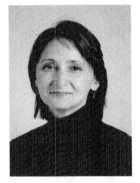

Sierra Farris, MA, MPAS, PA-C is a board certified Physician Assistant with master's degrees in both Clinical Neurology and Bioethics. Sierra is an ACSM Certified Exercise Specialist and incorporates her clinical exercise training into her medical care. She has extensive experience in the medical, surgical and rehabilitative treatment of individuals with movement disorders and has treated over 1000 people with deep brain stimulation across the United States. Sierra developed and continues to manage one of a few nationally recognized intensive troubleshooting clinics for people with unsatisfactory results from DBS and Sierra is one of a few national programming instructors. Sierra's research and publications focus on improving the lives of people living with DBS.

OTHER BOOKS OR CHAPTERS BY THE AUTHORS

DBS: A Patient Guide to Deep Brain Stimulation. A patient guide for people with tremor, dystonia and Parkinson's disease who wish to learn more or are already living with DBS.

Every Victory Counts. Essential information and inspiration for a lifetime of wellness with Parkinson's disease. Distributed by the Davis Phinney Foundation. A self-care guide focused on inspiration, and personal empowerment for all people wanting to take control of life with PD.

More Than a Mountain. Chronicles the first Parkinson's and multiple sclerosis expedition to Mt Kilimanjaro. The climber's stories filled with inspiration, fears, dreams, courage and compassion remind us all to redefine the possible. The authors served as the group's medical support.

TO BE RELEASED IN 2014

Healing Parkinson's: A Holistic and Integrative Medicine Approach. A comprehensive review of the scientific rationale and healing potential of complementary medicine and personal healing written to inspire wellness for all people living with Parkinson's disease.

CPSIA information can be obtained at www.ICGtesting.com
Printed in the USA
LVOW01s1923100714

393767LV00025B/810/P

9 781497 549647